THE MENTAL BREAKDOWN OF A NATION

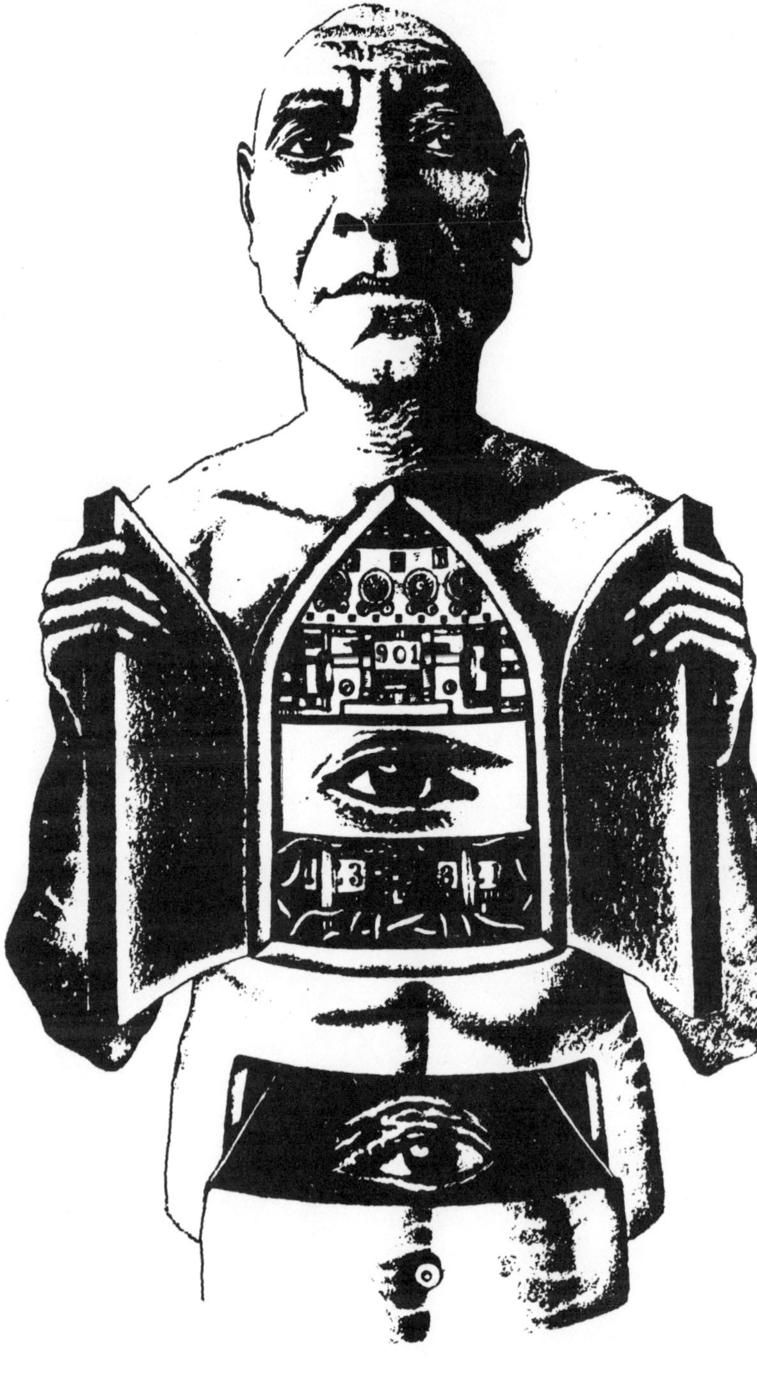
901

THE MENTAL BREAKDOWN OF A NATION

BY J. HERBERT FILL, M.D.

New Viewpoints, A Division of Franklin Watts, Inc. New York, 1974

Library of Congress Cataloging in Publication Data

Fill, J Herbert.
The mental breakdown of a nation.

Includes bibliographical references.
1. Social psychiatry—United States. 2. United States—Social conditions—1945- 3. Mental illness—United States. I. Title.
RC455.F48 362.2'04'220973 73-14739
ISBN 0-531-05353-9
ISBN 0-531-05559-0 (pbk.)

Printed in the United States of America
6 5 4 3 2 1

Cover design by Randall Deihl

Text design by Diana Hrisinko

CONTENTS

THE MENTAL BREAKDOWN OF A NATION

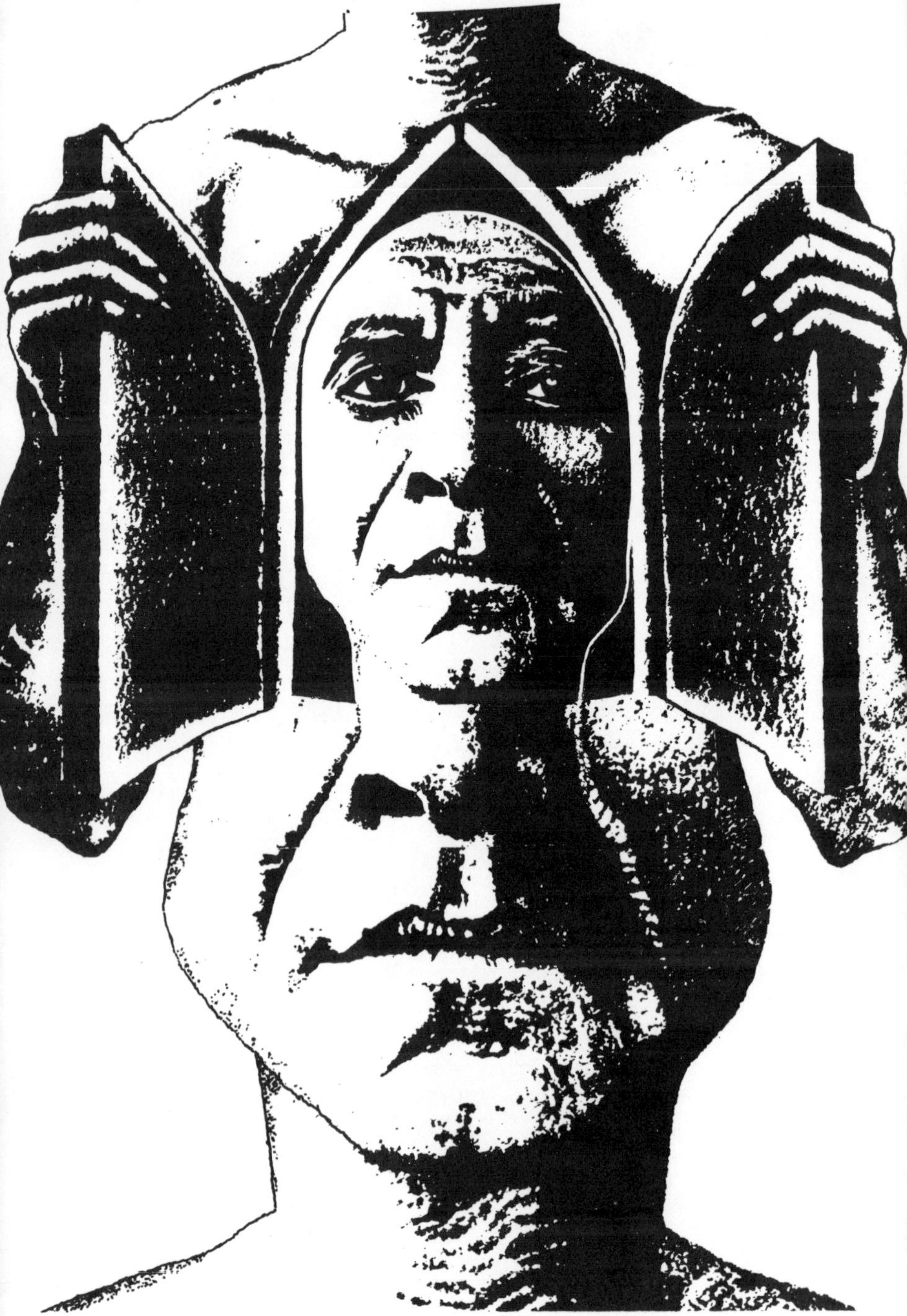

INTRODUCTION

There are in this country an estimated 4 million schizophrenics,[1] 4 million seriously disturbed children,[2] 6 million mentally retarded,[3] 9 million alcoholics,[4] and 10 million others suffering from severely disabling psychoneuroses, clinical depression, or antisocial and addictive disorders.[5]

This book does not deal with the clinical minority. The mental conditions that affect the *majority* of people are the real cause for alarm.

Ten years ago national and local surveys found approximately 80 percent of the adult population suffering from some form of mental disturbance.[6] Since then, admissions to psychiatric hospitals have increased annually, with our country's adolescents making up the fastest-growing segment of the inmate population. And new methods such as community psychiatry have been devised to treat the burgeoning numbers of patients outside hospitals.[7] Depressive conditions, from the subtle agonies of passive discontent to the cold gloom of suicidal despair, have now reached epidemic proportions. And everywhere we turn are the horrors of the rapidly rising mental disturbances labeled antisocial personality disorders: defacement, vandalism, shoplifting, fraud, theft, robbery, mugging, assault, rape, torture, kidnapping, hijacking, murder, and mass assassination.

We are surely witnessing the mental breakdown of a nation.

This book will describe how this mental breakdown, now accelerating at an alarming rate, is the tragic result of centuries of mental conditioning to a man-estranged world view.

Our mental destruction is upon us, and it rests largely on specific mental developments in the course of our history now aided, perpetuated, and exacerbated by modern education, technology, business, and mass communications that further deform and sicken our minds.

But there is a way out. This book proposes to shed the old world view that has determined our modern mental state. It suggests a process of mental reconstitution to achieve personal mental health. It also shows a way we can move toward the kind of social mental health that the largely unknown principles of mental health demand.

The operational plans of our major social institutions are the blueprints for insanity. Our old world view would carry these blueprints out to their final consequence with the power and momentum of an increasingly dehumanizing universe. The new view, dormant in the deepest recesses of our human subconscious, must be brought out into the light of consciousness. This new view will put a halt to the systematic destruction of our young and the new generations to come. There is still time to change the course that is rapidly leading us into the insane era of anti-man.

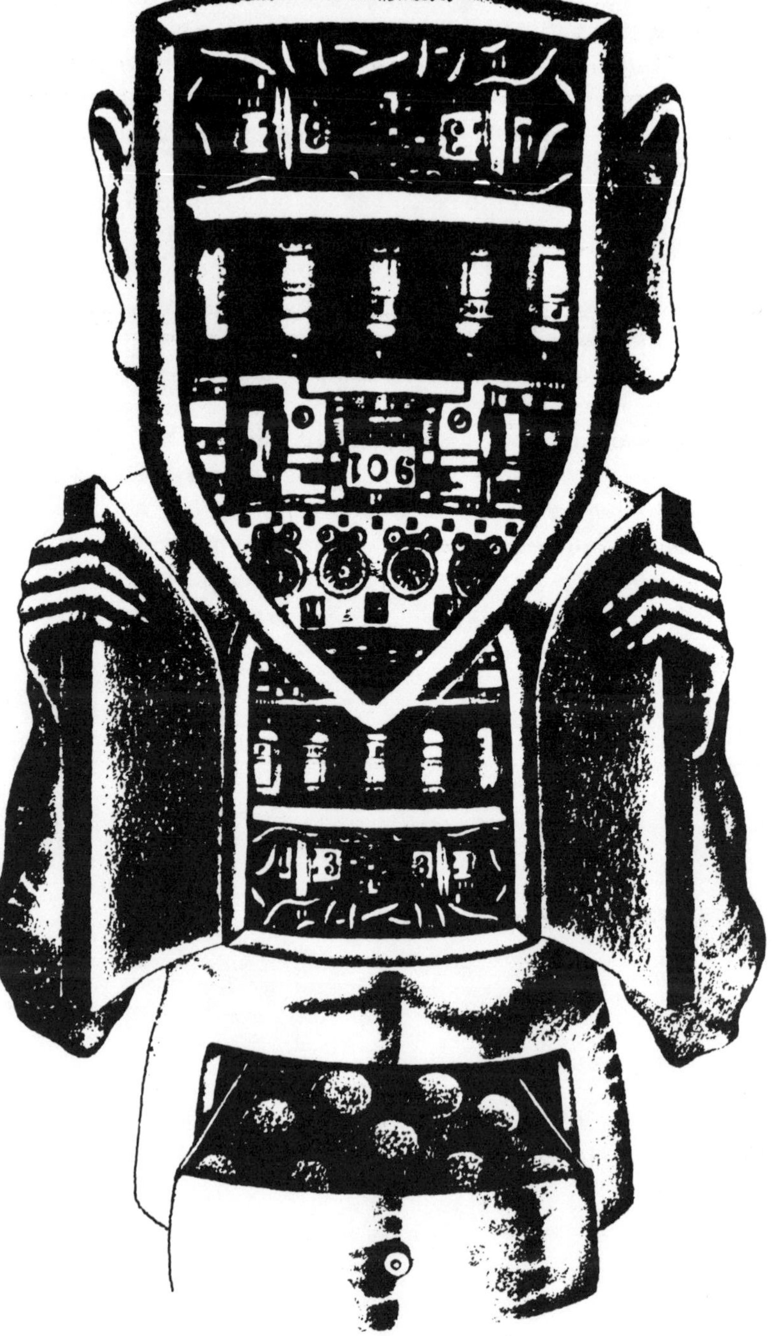
106

THE MAN-MADE CENTURY

"America, the Beautiful" was playing again. They were all there as usual, standing with hats in hand: the governor, the mayor, the board of trustees, the dignitaries, and the city officials all assembled in neat rows, this time to inaugurate the Brooklyn, New York, Children's Psychiatric Hospital. It was the sixth new children's psychiatric hospital to open this year.

The anthem was over and the governor rose. He looked out on the large gathering and began to speak with that characteristic self-confidence that put everyone at ease. The state was now building these facilities much more rapidly, thanks to the Health and Mental Hygiene Facilities Improvement Corporation and to the "terrific" advances in construction techniques. Treatment, too, had been "tremendously" improved by new drugs and behavior technology.

A rabbi followed him and spoke about the "blessing" visited upon the community by this new hospital and expressed "prayerful" hopes for the future of these children.

The chairman of the board of advisors, a wealthy industrialist and heavy contributor to mental care, closed on the high note of this being a truly magnificent example of government, business, clergy, and community all joining together to eradicate the evils of mankind and bring health and happiness to the three hundred unfortunate children who would soon find refuge and care in this wonderful new building.

Was this really such a happy occasion? To my mind it was a sad consequence of a much larger human tragedy that no one wanted to notice. Even more tragic, these dignitaries on the platform of social goodwill were the leaders of the very institutions *responsible for the mental de-*

velopments that have ultimately made such facilities necessary.

The bishop sitting next to the governor—who knows better than he how prescribed beliefs absolve us from thinking and consciousness, those human qualities that are essential in solving personal problems and maintaining good mental health?

The research scientist for the Department of Mental Hygiene sitting to my left is convinced that all truths now rest with science, forcing man to exclude feelings from a "true" view of himself and the world. But are not these same feelings the lifeblood of the whole, sane individual?

The chairman of the board also knows that our current use of technology substitutes human action and initiative with automation, causing a consequent loss of human will that almost guarantees a sick society.

And the government officials—certainly they have read the reports showing how the years of dehumanizing schooling they are enforcing are causing massive disabilities among millions of unwary children.

And what about myself? Surely as New York City mental health commissioner I must see the tragic paradox in striving to return disturbed children to a society that is itself mentally unhealthy!

Our children's basic mental functions were being destroyed piecemeal by our social institutions, and we, the protagonists of this gory and endless festival of "modern progress," were inaugurating yet another center to absolve ourselves from all responsibility for this systematic destruction of mental health.

The entire nation is like Brooklyn, New York. Professionals have convinced the federal government that two thousand comprehensive mental health centers blanketing the nation will solve our problem once and for all. For three hundred such centers "America, the Beautiful" has already been played, yet the casualties mount beyond measure. All over the country we are bandaging a few emotional cuts, yet with the very best of intentions we are actually expediting the mental slaughter of our children.

After the ceremony I headed back to my office in lower Manhattan. In the high morning sun I could see the ponderous towers of this man-made century, its "symbols of progress." The buildings I saw were states of mind materialized, their clashing designs and incongruous functions made of the same cloth as the minds that created them.

There was the stately Supreme Court with its ancient Roman image, featuring British-style jurisprudence now somehow translated into bail for the rich and jail for the poor. Adjacent to it was the Municipal Building, a tall caricature of the courtroom house where proof of a man's birth, existence, and even death rests with a computer. There was old City Hall, where today's youthful whiz kids futilely storm from wing to wing trying to find quick and cheap solutions to long-standing and expensive problems. Farther downtown were the cavernous estates of Wall Street with their ominous financial power . . . the windowless computer building of Bell Telephone, a contemptuous massive void in a city of human beings . . . and looming above them all, the latest symbol of social arrogance, the World Trade Center. I saw these powerful fragments of social functions—court, government, industry, finance—strewn about unrelated in shape and fashion, each one the expression of a fragment of our minds.

The city noise was its usual consistent roar. There seemed to be more litter than ever, tossed aside by people unaware of being caught up in the continual process of destroying their own world. Broken windows and graffiti on building walls testified to the mounting vandalism and willful defacement. The wary and unfriendly look on the faces of people around me was a harsh reminder of the rampant crime now threatening everyone with personal loss of life or property.

These are the crudest, most obvious signs of an insanely suicidal society. Like a colony of crazed animals that has lost its basic survival instincts, we are destroying ourselves in a fitful and mindless frenzy of hostility, destructiveness, and violence.

Everyone knows that something is dreadfully wong, but few see it as a particular, unhealthy mental configuration. We'd rather speak of social, political, economic, or other fragmented causes, all mere consequences of that mental state now destroying us.

As I walked through the city, agonizing questions came to my mind on whether my job had any real purpose or whether it was an insanity all its own. The city had become a huge greenhouse of florid, self-feeding abnormalities, and it was my job to supervise the mounting casualties of this greenhouse, either returning them restored to usefulness or removing them to avoid disrupting everyone else. Was there any sense in restoring people to a society that had no place for cultivation of the healthy human mind? At the moment I had to admit there was not.

Now it was midmorning. I looked out my office window to see Broadway filled with throngs of people laboriously winding their way to and from offices. The world view of generations was visible in their vacant faces and dogged determination.

Although their personal lives are in a mess, most

people still trudge to work, presumably to perform some useful function—not for themselves, of course, but for the company. They spend their time in offices dealing not with people but with paper, machines, typewriters, and computers. There is increasingly less room for creative, imaginative activity and more for detailed, predetermined, mechanical thinking.

The whole, feeling human being in us is now dominated by *intellect,* that mental faculty which through the centuries has grown far beyond its healthy limits. It is that faculty which demands that we *think think think* at the expense of everything else human within us. By not allowing feelings to "contaminate" an "objective" view, intellect has helped to create a dehumanized world view.

This murder of the intrinsic human being and the exclusive cultivation of intellect has reached frightening proportions in the 1970s. Our totally external approach to life has multiplied all the human problems that depend upon our feelings for others and our ability to act morally and independently.

We concentrate on external methods of birth control, but the largest reduction of births by far has arisen from the spontaneous change in people's attitude. This inner change has contained the population explosion in the United States, but it still remains a problem in underdeveloped countries where the external, scientific method is the *only* factor relied upon.

Modern medicine is considered to be one of the wonders of the world, but physical approaches such as surgery, medical technology, and laboratory techniques no longer aim at actual cure so much as they do at the removal of body parts or the elimination of symptoms. Except for antibiotics, most new drugs, such as steroids, antihistamines, tranquilizers, and analgesics, are almost entirely devoted to treating symptoms. The true concept of cure has been lost. More and more people do not live healthier lives; they are merely prevented from dying. There is indeed a technical but no *human* conception of what health is.

The threat of a nuclear holocaust has been in the back of our minds for decades. The threat presumably comes from within the "enemy's" mind, but our response, naturally, has been the building of bigger deterrents and antimissile systems.

There is nothing wrong with this pragmatic handling of a threat of war or of population problems, food production, pollution, poverty, illness—even mental illness. What is mentally abnormal and self-defeating is our single-minded insistence on purely external solutions. That simply is not enough to correct *human* problems.

It was almost 11:00 A.M. I had spent this part of the morning negotiating with the budget office to get a $200 annual salary increase for an employee. Now, a little later, I was asked to make my annual budget request for $160,000,000. I would have five minutes to present it.

The money was to operate psychiatric inpatient services in 26 hospitals and 106 mental health clinics in schools, courts, and prisons. I began to wonder what sort of "help" this is that no longer heals minds but simply returns patients to the society that caused their problems in the first place.

And what was sane behavior anyway? Was it "normal" to adjust to a stifling, intellect-drenched, dehumanized existence? Clearly, in these times to be fully adapted to society was in plain truth to be mentally *unhealthy*!

It was late morning when I returned to my office,

where there was a telegram on my desk signed by the Coordinating Committee of Employee Organizations—or the staff of the Board of Education:

> We, the 700 school psychiatrists, school psychologists, and school social workers in the Bureau of Child Guidance, along with the professional staff of the City Hospitals and the Coalition of Private Mental Health Agencies, vehemently object to the Department of Mental Health and Mental Health Retardation Services' latest proposals to restructure mental health services in the City. . . . (It) would jeopardize the Board of Education's ability to carry out its collective bargaining obligations and could result in endless litigation. . . .[1]

We had asked for negotiation of a contract indicating the time allotted for actual patient treatment. Of New York City's 1.3 million schoolchildren, 130,000 desperately needed help, yet the Rand Corporation had found that they received in direct service only 16 percent of the paid staff time of the Bureau of Child Guidance.[2] It was critical that services be substantially improved.

But would they? Judging from the telegram, the answer was no. The professional machine was shrieking at the merest hint of changes without even knowing what the changes might entail—or if they would be good or bad for the children. No one cared about the mental health of the children; the issue here was negotiation, and most likely the result of this conflict would be a watered-down compromise, a meaningless saving of faces . . . the inevitable non-solution of our times.

Mental health has much to do with why Johnny can't read. Of course, the expected dehumanized, external approach to the problem has been a cry for more schools, teachers, funds, and actual years of schooling. Yet these schools have become mental slaughterhouses where learning is rote, thoughts are misused and feelings are ignored, and, above all, children are being conditioned to disregard their own *human* development. This spirit in teaching is bound to induce pathology, and the public acceptance of the story related below is merely one example of a well-entrenched social insanity:

> This is the way Albert Shanker (present head of the United Federation of Teachers and a weekly syndicated columnist) used to teach: "If it takes four ounces of poison to kill a person, how many ounces would it take to kill your mother, your father, your sister and your brother?"—*Time,* May 29, 1972.

Pathology among pupils is on the rise, as children have begun to fight back in their own tragically self-destructive ways. The result is an educational system deteriorating into a process of management, disciplining, and policing. And the teachers, administrators, and school physicians aren't looking anymore at ways to handle the children's problems as much as they are trying to find a solution to their own. The "answer"? *Drugs.*

Drugs such as Dexedrine and Ritalin will quiet the increasing number of overactive children—an overactive child being one who cannot sit on a bench for five hours under bombardment by the most odious and repugnant teaching methods. Schools are now requiring an alarming number of children to take these behavior modification drugs, and as school attendance is mandatory by law, unwilling parents under threat of court procedure must now see their young forcibly drugged. There is an increasing number of horror stories telling of children begging to be taken off the required drugs, which are causing such side effects as loss of appetite, trembling, nightmares, exhaustion, and even mental breakdowns.

It was now almost noon. The director of a university psychiatric service had just called me to talk about a serious problem they were having with "soft drug" abuse by teen-agers. Would we fund a new type of clinic dedicated exclusively to treating this kind of condition? While I was listening to his request I leafed through the morning's stack of professional mail, noting the mountains of drug advertisements in the magazines, including the "most widely used behavior modifiers for problem pupils." I mentioned them to the caller, commenting on the connection between these medical journal ads and the need for new clinics such as the one he was proposing. "Well," he said, sighing, "someone [the drug industry] has got to finance our periodicals, don't you think?"

The government inflicts mental damage upon thousands of schoolchildren forced to take drugs, and then this same government finances clinics all over the country to treat drug abuse as a personal problem. It seems that our external approaches only breed bigger and more insoluble problems.

Government seems to be an eager party to even greater calamities. On my desk was a call from the president of the Board of Education for "computerized and automated school systems" with the objective of "imbuing each student with the habit of success." This actually means programming consoles at a level that "guarantees" success in following the prescribed routine.

The proposal continued: "The simple fact is that as mere reinforcing mechanisms, the teacher is out of date. If the teacher is to take advantage of the recent advances in the study of learning she must have the help of mechanical devices."

Teachers as mere "reinforcing mechanisms," reliance on mechanical devices—these make up the dream of the manipulator. He does not know of the intrinsic mental laws by which thought, feeling, and purpose grow or wither away in children. And this view, which turns a human being into a thing, is applauded by the scientific community and encouraged by the U.S. Department of Health, Education and Welfare, which is now spending millions to program the young electronically—regardless of the effects.

Soon these children may very well be in a "class of their own," as the electronics industry proudly advertises. That class will be inside a mental cubicle.

At this point it seemed as if I had spent my entire morning dealing with mental disruption and disaster related to educating "normal" children. I for one would rather learn from a possibly incompetent but human and full-blooded teacher than stare at ghosts on a screen conjured up by remote technicians who cannot or do not care what is happening to me.

It was now noon. I had been invited to see an old friend at the medical examiner's office, a place where it was tragically obvious that the casualties of our world view do not remain simply mental.

My friend showed me today's arrivals at the morgue. One youth revealed his way of dying by a streak of caked blood down his temple. There was a girl with the still, severe paleness of barbiturate death. Apparently no one had ever taught her to appreciate the beauty and dignity of that face. And farther down there was the young couple with the telltale pink patches of carbon monoxide death.

A world view estranged from human life had created mortal conflict for these young people. Man's mental suicide had sadly progressed to its ultimate physical conclusion.

Suicide is on the rise, and no solutions are at hand. Suicides are more difficult to prevent today because they are triggered by ever more superficial or seemingly irrelevant causes. An increasing number of young people are killing themselves because of parental criticism, failing grades, arguments over curfews, clothes.[3] The following suicide note left by a seventeen-year-old boy is sadly typical:

> Without a driver's license I have no car and without a car I have no social life so we might as well end it all right now.[4]

Emergency lines? They are usually too late for those who are serious. And it is difficult to quickly convince any prospective suicide victim of the value of his life as he stands on the window ledge after a lifetime in which his sense of his own value has been systematically destroyed. A true restoration of man's personal worth would do more to prevent suicide than all the hot lines, follow-up services, and hospital units put together.

Because they have no assurance of their individual value, students have relied on collective efforts to change institutions and society. This has brought death to the campus, and pointless violence and disruption, with no improvement in the situation whatever. Their ideas about change were shallow and lacking in true human values. Their agonized search for a more humanized society was tragically defeated by the prevailing world view so deeply entrenched inside them.

To appease their personal anguish and to obtain experiences society denies them, students often resort to drugs—yet another example of a manipulative, this time self-manipulative, solution to a human problem.

Students are also flocking to the social, life, and behavioral sciences—fields that are themselves the arch promoters of purely manipulative solutions. Showing unabashed contempt for the human aspects of man and denying even the possibility of his inner development, these fields try to change him in ways that are only external: drugs (psychotechnology), conditioning (behavior technology), a return to brain surgery, new electronic devices, electrode implantations. . . . Here our world picture is projected in its full horror: the mass insanity of physical and mental self-mutilation.

Students accept the idea that all human problems demand manipulation from without because they themselves are unwittingly manipulated. Their complete absorption in the present world view compels many of them to call for a "perfected" technology to solve all social problems. And this is exactly what the interests of technology want: no will or feelings needed—only intellect to respond. This advancing technology is just another step in the conditioning toward full mental passivity, toward an era in which there will be very little "human" about us.

I returned to my office in the early afternoon. There was a telephone message from a person I call the "lady of tranquillity." She periodically phoned to inquire about the effect the latest tranquilizer would have on her skin, always needing my assurance that her doctor was prescribing the right thing.

Her taking of tranquilizers had become second nature. She no longer observed her reactions to life but to the tranquilizer and her derived satisfaction from "doing well by it."

Housewives are the largest consumers of tranquilizers. It is probably no coincidence that they are also the segment of society most dependent on their family and the surrounding world; their inner happiness is most likely to rely on external gratification and approval. In a sense, we are all this way. We have allowed society's institutions, conventions, establishment, and political structures to dominate our lives, for we have given them the power to determine how we see ourselves. In our madness we have become conditioned to accept corporate, governmental, ideological, and belief systems as somehow more valid than ourselves. But good mental health and true happiness must come from within—from a person's understanding and appreciation of his own individual worth.

At 2 P.M. I took part in a public hearing of the Health and Hospitals Corporation in the Bellevue Nursing School Auditorium in New York City. Here was an opportunity for people to complain about the services and propose new ways to improve the care. But the crowd was in an aggressive, contemptuous, derisive mood, and a rumble of chattering interspersed with catcalls and insults prevented everyone from hearing the president's version of what was wrong.

The afternoon was filled with shouting and occasional fistfights. Power, jobs, salaries, promotions, staff privileges—these were the most vocal and persistent themes. A Black member of the board rose to speak for more minority representation in high executive positions; a union leader emphasized the rights of the workers; another spokesman called for community control in health services. Not to be outdone, a Chinese stood up and exclaimed, "Do not forget the Chinese!"

This was a paranoid jumble of clashing interests, entirely unrelated to the improvement of human health for all. It was social sickness in full view, a spectacle of complete social disintegration amid unbridled drives.

By adopting the strategies of manipulatory "solutions" and by its crude exhibition of pressure, threats, and intimidations, the public itself was ironically driving a machine—a public corporation—into further dehumanization. By forcing it to respond to all their divergent needs, by making it promise to give everyone "a piece of the pie," the protesters diverted the corporation's attention from the individual patients' (human) needs. The whole man had once again been squeezed out of the picture.

It was now late afternoon. I returned to my office to find it filled with angry people. The staff and the mentally retarded charges of one of our contract agencies were sitting on my desk and tables; papers were flying or being scribbled on everywhere. What did I have against these poor mentally retarded children? Why did I continue to deprive them of their care? The staff representatives, obviously not caring about the lesson in aggression they were imparting to these youngsters, wanted me to commit myself in writing to hiring of two unqualified people, or I would not be permitted to leave the office. To meet the next morning when my staff was available to assess the situation was unacceptable to them until a diplomatic police officer listed the number of charges that would be lodged against them unless . . .

The heads of this agency had actually *used* the sick

to promote personal interest, a fully accepted practice in the modern technique of confrontation. The disabled had been nothing but a pawn for the plays for power of the even sicker self-proclaimed helpers. This extends to inflated budget requests, union demands, community boards, assorted health associations, legislators on pre-election tours, and the flashy "exposés" presented by the news media. All organizations tend rapidly to become self-serving as they operate within our world picture.

The victims have become the victimizers. Calls for societal change, change in the corporate state and in the structures of establishments, institutions, and the Church, have all been in vain. They only illustrate the continuing implicit denial of man's essential reality as an individually responsible entity.

Our current world picture clearly indicates no intrinsic interest in human problems, but rather an interest in the usefulness of people in keeping society running smoothly in the direction *determined by that dehumanized world picture.*

The Joint Commission on Mental Health of Children had this to report to the President of the United States:

> It should be emphasized that fostering the development of human beings in this country is a means to an end—a means to stem the increasing numbers of people who have no meaningful role in society. . . . In our children lie our future and our hope for the fulfillment of our national goals.[5]

Here service is not conceived as helping the individual on his own terms, but simply activating him to serve a "national goal" set by our own views of life. To be able to attend school, hold down a job, raise a family—most organized care-giving efforts aim basically at these goals of social usefulness.

This is a dangerous proposition. It is saying that *man exists only as a function*—as an exchangeable part in the larger machine of society. This depersonalized view has little to do with human development, and as such it can only lead us further down the path of mental destruction.

An attitude is taking hold that all conceivable public services should be expanded to cover "all service needs" of the population. This view, of course, inspires individuals, groups, neighborhoods, politicians, and government officials to become "aware" of every new "need" that is unfulfilled and even to proclaim new needs wrapped in words such as "progress," "quality of life," and "rights." This substitution of ever-expanding services for human self-help efforts is further evidence of a world view that encourages dependency, dehumanization, and continuing disability. Once again, the whole human being is ignored.

People of the "communities" have caught on to the notion that they are nothing without power, prestige, and money. This accurate reflection of current world views has produced a new phenomenon that has brought orderly, productive government and positive change to a virtual halt.

Community groups have sprung up everywhere to function as small human machines. Often run by ambitious, ruthless leaders (who go on to greener pastures as soon as they have intimidated governments into giving them better-paying jobs as "concerned experts" in community affairs), they are the latest expression of social distrust and manipulation.

Rather than connoting real interest and effort, community involvement has become a euphemism for *demand.*

Questions of "representation," policy-making, power, control, and the clamor for "executive" jobs seem to be the real issues—not the sorely needed projects that pressure, blackmail, and threats often block before they are begun. Any improvement is elusive, and most neighborhoods in most cities are actually deteriorating.

What is really deteriorating is the mental health of the community members who pursue these harmful practices. As more groups are seduced into demanding advantages over the needs of others, we are moving even closer to a social hell of innumerable conflicts and rifts that tear apart our social fiber. Cloaked in the guise of concern, involvement, and rights, these antisocial forces of manipulatory intellect and publicly sanctioned drives are destroying our communities. The encouragement of spurious needs and demands and the rhetoric of rights as they are exploited today only spur more controls as rising demands create a tightening of benefits. This conflict between misguided demands and reactive control can only spread and progressively deepen human strife.

We demand the earth, but our own immense human needs are often considered last, when they are considered at all. In the past few years only $10 million of $62 million appropriated by Congress for child mental health was permitted to be spent; meanwhile $250 million went to Lockheed, hundreds of millions to the Penn Central Railroad, and billions to highway construction. Big corporate demands, political needs, and the desires the man in the street has had foisted upon him are obviously valued above truly human needs. Is there any other explanation why no community in this country provides an acceptable standard of service for emotionally disturbed youth? [6] People actually have a low priority in our society.

When we do attempt to deal with our human problems, our external approach usually defeats us. How to handle lead poisoning? Why, the most effective, cheapest, and quickest way, of course: in a simple mechanical process, test the children; get the positive reactors into hospitals; board up the walls of the lead-laden ghetto apartments; then return the children to them when the work is completed.

What this method completely ignores is the *child* who suffered the poisoning the first place. His eating of paint is really an emotional disturbance related to neglect and lack of supervision. Removing a three- to six-year-old to a hospital results in psychic trauma, the institutionalization syndrome, withdrawal apathy, and functional retardation since their stay there is usually protracted. The child may never recover. But this is the sadly typical result when we ignore the inner human problem.

The dehumanizers are all around us. The National Institute of Mental Health actually believes that it serves society when it supports behavioristic calls for social control and mass conditioning, just as the U.S. Department of Health, Education and Welfare feels it is "modernizing" education when it supports electronic "teaching" with utterly no thought given to the mental effects on children. Intellect can think of man only as a function, and the result is his dehumanization.

It no longer suffices to speak of dehumanization in a generalized fashion. This statement of self-estranged *thinking* shows that it is a tragic experience for each individual:

> I had a family, a house, a car, a career all cut out for me. What was now missing was to live all this. So far, I played the game as it was played, but made no rules. The rules had been set by someone unknown and the rules made the game. I kept playing and made all the

> right moves, as if my life depended on it all. It did. My "playing" life depended on someone or something unknown that did not care. I want to be in on my own life. I want to act like me, not some plastic person.[7]

This anguished human being felt a loss of self-experience, with a consequent loss of ability to relate to external reality. This is a common condition, although most of us are not aware of such cracks in our self-image. We do not know ourselves.

Another case history showed self-estranged *feelings*:

> I'd like to change the whole world. I don't like anybody, really, least of all myself. I want so much to be loved, but I would never believe it could happen. I spend most of my energies not feeling something fully myself but preventing myself from having certain feelings. To be safe from myself is all I am asking, is all I am working on. But I keep generating this hostility directed at no one in particular, and I freeze. Most of my life is spent not in *living* feelings, but in *screening* them out and into oblivion. That is so because the feeling I would want to have I consider harmful. I must forever escape them. I simply couldn't take any more harm, I would come apart.[8]

These are the so-called neuroses that freeze us into an emotional "set" of fear and hostility. Anxiety and rigidity, fixations and obsessions now affect a vast majority of people.

It was 5 P.M. I had one last meeting, and it was the one I dreaded most. I knew my position had no chance to succeed, but I had to make it clear in order to know for certain whether our present world view was so dehumanized that it would continue to allow the killings of hundreds of living beings.

The meeting was not on legal abortion—that had already become New York State Law—but on its twenty-four-week limit. Hundreds of abortions around the sixth month of pregnancy had actually resulted in live babies, which were then dumped into trash cans whimpering or left to die. I requested that we work to reduce the time limit. Did the mother always know the time of conception? How about the rights of a living human being who was alive on earth just as his mother was? Could he be put to death "legally" without a trial? What would be the mental effects on the mother if she knew that her aborted fetus became a newborn baby dying in the garbage? What about the demoralization among doctors and nurses? There was a silent cold stare in response to my questions. I had visions of New York as a single great machine made up of cold, clammy, mindless human parts operating by the book of instructions while the discussion drifted into statistics and press releases about thousands of abortions . . . no deaths. . . .

The concept of being a mere by-product of nature has dehumanized us. It has wasted our minds and mental energy. We have indeed become a social organism that is dangerous to itself and others, and this is the legal definition of insanity.

We are all engaged in a struggle to maintain personal sanity these days, for our society leaves no room for anyone to be an exception:

> I had never had any questions about my sanity, but lately I have had some sudden and frightful doubts when I realized that I myself and the world out there did not really go together. Besides, was that world

real? Was I? I only knew that I felt utterly suspended in a kind of psychic void with no support anywhere. If that were so, I thought that nothing could make any difference any longer, nothing at all. There was no place to go in that kind of phantom world that I felt I could sink into anytime. . . . Actually, I was already sinking, and had been from the days of my childhood. I remember the relentless schooling that seemed to choke me with undigestible foreign matter. It was constantly implied that I could only be "right" if filled with all that stuff, and everyone in college or even the newspapers or T.V. just kept filling me up with the same old things. I could have turned off most of it, at least at home, but there was also that obligation to be "with it." And so I kept eroding my inner strength, surrendering more controls to the outside and kind of liking the benefits. I had lost not only the sense, but the ability of self-mastery. In short, I had become like a sponge, soaking up everyone else's words and sensations which were not really their own but those they thought they should have.[9]

This agonized statement by one of my patients sadly typifies the loss of identity we are all suffering. Each one of us must struggle to discover his own reality as a deeply experienced fact at the center of his being, and to see the world on his own terms. If we do not, we shall some day witness the total annihilation of personal man. When that day comes, we will no longer be able to survive as human beings.

The day was coming to a close. The patients in hospitals or visiting clinics and therapists were desperately trying to recover their humanity and wholeness. But what troubled me more was the insanity I had seen spreading among the "healthy" people.

There was the inauguration of the Brooklyn Children's Psychiatric Hospital, and the knowledge that even the scenes filmed by those television cameras would be sandwiched in the news between *Circle of Fear* and *Let's Make a Deal.* I could still hear the insults and obscenities hurled at the corporation's meeting. I had met the fatal depressions of the young in the city morgue. I had viewed the antisocial practice of manipulating patients on behalf of vested interest. I had heard people ignore live abortions in order to get good publicity. Every event in my day had demonstrated how our behavior has clearly become insanely dangerous to ourselves and others. We function in the illusion that we are sane, but we continue to violate the crudest principles of mental health.

And I was one of the perpetrators. Each day my position allowed me to help turn the wheels of the bureaucratic machines that grind man's humanity into oblivion. If I really wanted to come to grips with the human problems behind our institutionalized insanity, I would have to step outside my office and apply all my energies to understanding the root causes of our trouble. Consequently, my last act of the day was to submit my resignation as New York City commissioner of Mental Health and Mental Retardation Services.

On my way home, the lighted city appeared almost serene. I had occasion to think ruefully of other dangers that were besetting this still-great city from without, intruding into the minds of its people.

Some of our prominent scientists have taken it upon themselves to make our struggle for sanity even more difficult. Intensely interested in the domain of ethics, religion, humanism, behavior, human affairs, and man himself, they have taken old concepts applicable to matter only and applied them to human beings. Worse, they think themselves fit to discourse on the whole man by comparing him to one small fragment of nature.

Konrad Lorenz, well-known ethologist, knows his animals well, so he concludes that animal traits make up all of man. Lionel Tiger and Robin Fox, respected paleontologists, imply that "man's mind development appears inextricably a by-product of spine lengthening and buttock expansion." [10] B. F. Skinner, expert in the conditioning of lower animals, derives a picture of man and an entire design of culture from the changes of rate of responses to stimuli of the rat. Jacques Monod, eminent geneticist, observes once more that genes come about by chance and proceed by necessity, and then concludes that everything there is to know about man is globular protein.

On the basis of comparable scientific evidence one could state with equal omniscience that all our social problems will be solved by placing windmills at strategic locations all over this country.

The windmills of intellect are being introduced into our life sciences, our mental health professions, and our schools to justify further the old world picture by new "scientific" somersaults.

Meanwhile, to look at this city, this entire country, is to see it screaming, bleeding, dying the insane self-destructive death of a mind turned against itself. It is not only the collective scream of the killed, raped, and mugged; it is the inner, silent outcry of those being destroyed from within. It is most urgent that there be a new view of our world and that there be meaningful solutions to human problems, solutions unfettered by the dehumanized thoughts we have so tragically allowed to develop through the centuries. We need to view the whole man, and we need human ways to counteract what is a human catastrophe.

How did the tragedy of today happen? How did the role of intellect, consciousness, feeling, will, and drives change over time to create the present insanities of our social existence, our "modern" life, our education, and technology? What were the mental steps in history that brought us to this crisis? What exactly is the nature of our present world picture? How can we save ourselves?

A day in the office directing the mental health department of a modern American city flung these pressing questions at me and at least offered a few clues.

One thing was certain. If man has the immense heritage he has, and if his mind has passed through such manifold and varied transformations, then he must be a being of great value. One could stumble and err in describing his tragic, complex mental change, but there could be no easy way out of flippant explanations or solutions. For something terrible has happened and is happening not only to nature but to man in this man-made century.

THE SCHOOL: AN EDUCATION IN INSANITY

More than any other institutions, it is our schools that contribute to the deepening mental breakdown of our society. Through the science and technology that education deifies, modern schooling denies the child his being, destroys his faculty of thinking, vitiates his feeling, obliterates his will, floods him with festering personal and social neuroses, and fosters fearsome antisocial disorders that are assailing ever-larger segments of our population. It is truly in our schools that the old, man-estranged world picture is perpetuating itself with disastrous consequences.

The Invalidation of the Child

Although there has been effusive criticism of the schools from parents, educators, psychologists, community leaders, politicians, unions, and even the electronics industry, it seldom expresses concern for the child himself. No one points to the grueling, mentally harmful effects of schooling—its shattering of the spirit of those children already dispirited by poor, broken, or disrupted homes; its crushing of those who cannot endure its procrustean and crippling methods.

Few questions are raised about the schools' role in the skyrocketing drug abuse, destructiveness, and criminality among the young. Nor are the critics voicing alarm at recent research findings that report that in Manhattan alone only 12 percent of the juvenile population can be considered mentally healthy.

The welfare of the child is rarely the concern of the schools' critics. Rather, the complaints have to do with the particular stakes various groups feel they have in the educational system.

The electronics industry wants a market for its educational aids. Parents want disciplined children. Politicians desire visibility. Psychologists are only interested in pupil "adjustment." Community leaders are after power. The union is foremost concerned with the privileges of its teacher members, privileges that make it possible for a teacher to face a once-in-a-lifetime exam with no need to update knowledge; to have tenure based on time, not performance; never to be dismissed for reasons short of malfeasance; to return to teach after many years of absence for the sole purpose of obtaining a pension. In all these demands the child appears as an inanimate commodity subject to wholely extraneous arrangements. He has no rights of his own, for a school's opening, closing, teaching, orientation, goals, and architectural design usually have nothing to do with children but rather with a myriad of concerns that are a reflection of interests based upon our "scientific" world view. In our profound collective lack of interest in true education, we continue to deny our humanity as well as our mental abilities.

The Destruction of Thinking

The teacher was saying to the eighth graders, "All we need to do is always have the facts straight and use them. Most of these facts are still quite beyond our control. Science will get them under control; technology will get them to work for us."

This is the kind of "thinking" our modern schools are supporting. It totally excludes the ability or interest to know one's self, to think independently, and to relate knowledge to human obligations. All experience is downgraded to a search for facts and all joy of discovery to a search for utilization of what is discovered. Thinking is actually dissipated into basic thoughtlessness, and consciousness is altogether ignored. This is intellect at work, and it pervades the education of the child from his earliest years in the classroom.

Our worship of intellect has allowed us to "hurry" children in their education, often with disastrous results. In our relentless pressure for early *conceptualization,* we ignore the powerful learning impulses of active imagination in preschool children, and the need for mental imagery for those of the early grades. As it is difficult for the young child to form concepts, the result is usually frustrating failure. This can immunize the child against free and spontaneous ideas. Later, thinking abilities will also be compromised by their association with stress. Under such conditions IQ's will tumble in the course of the first school years.

Yet once children *can* handle concepts, they are fed "facts" unrelated to meanings, feelings, or personal experiences. The facts are therefore indigestible. The school tries to overcome this natural reaction by rote memorizing that turns off a child's own thinking further and heightens his passive acceptance. At this point, thinking has become *indoctrination.*

When concepts are presented, they are often little more than facts themselves, to be memorized but never pondered. This approach to ideas and the plethora of factual information children are forced to absorb leave no time or energy for reflective thought and degrade their minds into mere containers. They no longer think about facts but assume these facts, or indoctrinations, to be thinking itself. Children soon realize that they don't exist by virtue of their thinking and that their personal consciousness has no value. They exist only as a function, and even that remains to be confirmed by measurable means—mainly by misuse of grading.

This kind of education trains children to become sophists. They learn to think what is convenient or pleases, not what might be true or what might lead to personal mental development. The very self of the child is lost, and the essence of thinking is destroyed.

The Vitiation of Feelings

The American educator John Dewey once observed that a child lives largely by emotions in and out of schools—whether he is allowed to do so or not. It would follow, therefore, that a child's emotional state holds the key to his educational success. How he feels determines his openness and attitude toward seeking knowledge, his co-operation, his initiative, and his enthusiasm. Feelings are indeed the wellspring of a child's learning ability.

Unfortunately, schools tend to ignore the child's feelings or, more precisely, ignore the feeling child as a whole being. They destroy the very foundation of the child's interest, enthusiasm, and motivation, which is the heart and substance of any true education. Children are taught as if their feelings did not, or should not, exist. In fact, feelings are considered a nuisance in our intellectually dominated schooling. As a protective reflex, the child gradually learns to deny his own spontaneous feelings, automatically "checking" his emotional reactions to see if they are safely within the implied margins approved by the institutions.

> At one point in my life I realized that most of my feelings were not fully and truly my own. They seemed to be experiences force-fed into me by standards my

> parents and schools set up. They had nothing at all to do with my own personal feelings but I came to accept them as my own. Now all my feelings seem strange and painful even when I think I am happy.[1]

If the child's own feelings are suppressed or considered "invalid," his private feelings about the world become loaded with resentment. Of all insults, it is this personal exclusion of self that offends a child most in life, converting his potentially positive emotions into aggressive or self-destructive hostility.

Exposure to school during these formative years will condition the child negatively toward knowledge, life, success, and mastery. More specifically, it will tend to exacerbate inferiority feelings, self-defeating reactions, escapism, dishonesty, apathy, or frank emotional disturbances. The latter in turn will translate into mental backwardness or antisocial reaction.

It is no accident that vandalism is on the rise, having risen in estimates from millions to hundreds of millions of dollars in the past few years in New York City alone. Buildings everywhere have been defaced with indelible spray paint. Secret names and numbers sprawled upon buses and subway cars indicate the writers' search for self-confirmation in a purely external and publicly destructive form. Classroom behavior itself clearly shows how rejected and ignored feelings turn into this sick aggression.

> The boys in my class found a new pastime when the teacher's out: running around the room wrecking everything in sight. . . . Actually, I don't even think they're really enjoying themselves but since it's so easy to do when the teacher isn't there, they just go ahead and do it.[2]

If schools are not rejecting feelings outright, they are eliciting *negative* feelings.

In some schools a feeling of detachment is promoted as a matter of routine:

> I feel like I'm going to burst with excitement when I'm very involved with something during class—maybe a chemistry experiment—but I have to stop immediately when the bell rings. That's the signal to close up your brain to chemistry until 1:45 P.M. the next day. So I've given up on school. I can learn better when I'm out, just reading and exploring things on my own. I'm physically in school every day, but I remove myself as much as possible. It's like splitting myself in half.[3]

And there is fear itself, a sinister promoter of neurotic self-estrangement: "The school system is based upon fear. Students are taught from the outset that they should be afraid of having certain things happen to them: bad grades, punishment from authorities, humiliation, ostracism, "failure," antagonizing teachers and administrators are all things that terrify students as they enter first grade. These fears which school officials use as a lever from elementary school through high school to establish and maintain order and obedience, have horribly destructive effects: they may be reflected in extreme nervousness, terror, resentment, withdrawal, alienation. . . ."[4]

And children are taught to hate:

> June 17—*Last Day.* Yesterday all our teachers who screamed at us all year said we'd been lovely students—we'd brightened up their lives. What bull! They hate us, just as we hate them, but now that school's over they're so happy they don't care what

they're saying. They say things they don't really mean. SCHOOL'S OVER!!![5]

The assistant principal said today, "I am a rough man and a hard man, so you'll be treated roughly and you'll have to be hard too! . . ." One of these days I'm not going to do anything and teach some other people that I can be mean too. It might be soon. I still haven't learned anything. When will I? We can't even open our mouths here. What is this, a communist country —the kids and teachers can't speak their piece? Can't stand one, single kid in this stupid idiotic place. If I have to kill myself, I will get out of here.[6]

Children are creatures with feelings. By ignoring those feelings or promoting negative ones in order to push ahead with a child's "intellectual development," our schools have spawned mental deformities beyond anyone's wildest nightmares. Inferiority complexes, self-defeating reactions, escapism, dishonesty, apathy, destructiveness—these are the horrendous mental consequences of a modern education. And worst of all, the children are not learning anything. Nor can we expect them to, until we recognize that feelings are as much a valid part of the educational experience as they are a force within children themselves.

The Obliteration of Will

There is still another area of the mind that is adversely affected by schooling. It is the sphere of our willpower, a mental area notoriously remote from our awareness, and greatly misunderstood.

Will is usually confused with drives, instincts, or impulses. It is none of these, but an ability comparable to musculature—a basic mental faculty that is strong or weak depending on exercise. Only our own exertion can increase muscle power; if someone else were to flex any one of our limbs a thousand times a day without any effort on our own, our muscles would remain as flaccid as ever. *This is what is being done to our wills in our school life.*

Teachers, unfamiliar with the nature of will, continually suppress or compel rather than guide or stimulate the child's muscles of will, with the consequence that this vital mental ability is weakened or destroyed.

And the schools themselves institutionally ignore the importance of will, preferring to prescribe to the dictates of behaviorism to develop the child. This external approach usually causes the child's will to wane, having been crushed under the undue regimentation and control.

Schools not only destroy the child's will; they encourage him to surrender it. The student who passively follows directions, who unquestioningly listens to his teacher, and who submissively adapts himself to course content becomes a "success" in the system, for it is he who is the school's desired end product.

From a student newspaper:

> Students who have been passive for twelve years in the face of authority will be superbly fitted for colleges that are based on submission to authority and scholarly pecking orders. They fit very well in an economic system based on submission to bureaucratic organization, mass production, and cut-throat economic self-interest.[7]

Through such basic passivity, which pervades all of schooling, the ability for self-generated action is killed.

One result is the children's much bemoaned apathy and unwillingness to work.

In and out of school, the fate of these children will be much the same as that of GI's released after years of regimentation in the army, where every detail of their daily lives had been determined. Or the fate of those Chinese refugees who, after a lifetime of regimentation on the mainland, took a nighttime swim from Canton to Hong Kong. Or that of any prisoner released from long-term detention. They feel lost and helpless when they suddenly find themselves within a free society, where in order to survive they must suddenly exert individual initiative and engage in self-determined action and perseverance.

The children emerging from our schools are will-cripples. Many of them try to prolong some study arrangement, or they substitute for school an establishment that offers security, job protection, clearly defined tasks, non-involvement, and all possible fringe benefits for the least possible effort. They have learned well how to please authority and how to act in order to be "successful."

One of school's poisoned gifts will be the twisting of our minds into the delusion that these benefits give life meaning. Only after graduation will we be free to learn that meaning rests on our *own* accomplishments. But for many it will be too late to approach life in this mentally healthy way.

School has made our mental abilities become external demands. Inner being has been preempted—a stunning blow to our mind, our mental health, and our very humanity.

School-Induced Neuroses

The basic modern concepts governing our schools create their own pathology. Viewing education as a compartmentalized activity separate from other activities of life such as work, entertainment, human development, and life purpose, they aid in the *fragmentation of a child's personality.*

Promulgating the acquisition of knowledge and skills at the expense of the development of the entire personality has resulted in a *child's mental breakdown.*

And the treatment of thought not as a skill of the total intelligence, but only as a passive absorbtion of knowledge, has created *children with a limited, preconceived picture of the world.*

Everywhere we look, our schools' institutionalized insanity is contributing to the neuroses of our young.

The schools have a basic contempt for the human being, whose unpredictability is considered a risk. It is this mental orientation that has led to so much imposed docility, such meager faith in individual performance, and such joylessness and repression of spontaneity.

The obsession with force-feeding the three R's as quickly as possible has led to passive children who surrender their personalities to the system for the system's sake. The schools are not concerned with really developing a child's love of learning; rather, the ideal pupils would be puppets who would be released to form a puppet society. One student described it this way:

> I've learned through experience that rule number one for school survival is Don't Question Anything. Don't ask about rules, don't question why you have to study about ancient Egypt. Because *they* don't like it. But I do what I'm told, carrying out orders like a puppet on a string, pulled this way and that by the teachers. In school I'm not *me* anymore. The trouble is, sometimes I begin to feel like a machine even out of school. I mean, when I'm left on my own with some free time, I

don't know what to do with myself. It's like I'm waiting for someone to come along and *tell* me: Read this book. Write that letter. I guess I've gotten so used to dictatorship, I'm lost when I'm free.[8]

This child has come to need the strings as much as he hates them. He has acquired a school-induced conflict that will harm his career, his relationships with people, his very mental health. He has learned to hate his task, or do nothing. He has learned to function by not being himself. He has learned to be *neurotic.*

Even if teachers are not imbued with the rigid, depersonalized philosophy of the schools, they are often helpless to change the situation. Although they might wish to have a freer, more spontaneous classroom, they fear they will lose their audience unless they enforce the rules they often view with distaste. And if they initiate their own small but meaningful reforms, they will be sure to hear the buzzing gossip of other teachers, the condemnation of such "heretical" procedures by principals, or criticism by parents or the community.

It has been mentioned before that the frustration of failure produces tremendous aggression or ruthlessness in normal children. By this route, the "slow" child will be led into acting "abnormally" more quickly than others and will then, upon the teacher's demand, be transferred to sections often referred to as "discipline classes," "custodial classes," "jungle classes," "zoos," or classes "one can forget about as far as teaching is concerned."

Children can become absolutely neurotic about their intellectualism. If they cannot succeed at being intellectual, some children will at least try to imitate being so:

Among the fourth grade classes at one school . . . the teachers of the three slow classes refer to their

> charges as "crazy," "the worst kids in the grade," and as lacking imagination because, in one teacher's words, "they don't even want to draw." No, they don't want to, they prefer to write. They even prefer to write something like "I must sit in my seat" a hundred times rather than draw.[9]

They would rather fail at intellectualism than succeed at anything else.

One of the major causes of children's neuroses is one of the least suspected but most insidious practices of schools: the systematic cultivation of competition among students.

Competition is alleged to stimulate performance. It does not, however, foster self-initiated accomplishment, the kind of initiatives the child will need in independent adult life; it simply compels "response" performance. Competition conditions the child to think that his being consists in function alone, while it is the building of his *own* initiatives that is true preparation for adult accomplishment. Once again, the schools reveal their ignorance of the mental facts of life and their cynicism toward whole men.

A complaint from a top high school athlete:

> The teachers slap my back, the principal even calls me in his office to talk about the game I won, the kids look up to me. But they're not fooling me. They don't really care about me as a person, only about the glory I give the school. The teachers aren't allowed to fail me because they need me on the football team. So I'm passed every year but I don't know nothing and they don't even try to help. I'm seventeen now. I'm too small to make it in pro sports and forget about college. After I graduate it'll probably just be downhill all

the way. Then they'll see that I'm really a nobody underneath it all. And I have those teachers to blame for keeping me a hero who doesn't know what anything's about.[10]

A competitive society is an immature society. One can only compete for power, prestige, and possessions. It is impossible to compete for one's being, its quality, its scope, its power, for that is a matter of achievement within oneself. Competition is a perverted form of passivity in which we ourselves never change and are recognized only as a reflection of what we are required to do. Introduced intentionally into schools, competition is the seed for a dehumanized universe. A competitive society is a dehumanized society; the fiercer the competition, the less room for overall *human* development.

It is ironic that even when children do not become neurotic through our schools, their "healthiness" is often expressed in destructive ways. When children do make an effort to learn, for example, and the knowledge they acquire consists of mere facts devoid of meaning, their dissatisfaction will often cause them to rebel. The morning vomiting so common among young children is another attempt to resist an unhealthy educational environment. So no one succeeds in our schools, whether they be classified as neurotic or healthy. If our educational system continues to exist in its present form, the loathing children feel against the schools will never be overcome. They will instead proceed to destroy those schools. Some have already started.

Manipulation as the Answer

Educational neuroses are festering, and the aversion most children have for school is almost taken for granted these days. And instead of seeking ways to develop teaching as an art that places the child at the center of its attention, there is a constant search for new methods of manipulation. The pupils learn quickly to imitate that very manipulation:

> You might call me an educational con man. I know how to give the teacher what he wants even though my mind is a million miles away thinking about the weekend coming up or whatever. It's easy, no secret formula, practically everyone does it. You just look the teacher in the eye when he's droning on about something, nodding here and there when he pauses, smiling or frowning when he does. It looks like you're oh so *intensely* involved. The teacher will love you for it and at the same time the game frees your mind to go in your own direction. It's failproof. I picked it up early in grade school and I've been doing it ever since.[11]

If the student won't play the con game, the educators only seek new shortcuts to manipulate him. The usual solution seems to be: let's pretend they haven't got a mind.

William C. Morse of the University of Michigan highlights the current "conflict" within education:

> Some advocates cling to a simpleminded hope that affection and acceptance will conquer all; others are just as certain that the only way to manage recalcitrant youth is to get tough and kick them out when they do not respond.[12]

Management by primitive or manipulative conditioning, a long-term practice in schools, is now being elevated to a science called behavior modification. This institutionalized cruelty, administered in ways the child will accept and ultimately embrace, is being justified as a method that has objective value as a means to an end. The end, purported to be for the good of the child, will be "good" for him only because it adapts him to the world dictated by our particular world view.

The crude reward-punishment reinforcements practiced have not improved education. Being grossly inadequate for our times, they have led only to rebellion in today's student body. They fail, too, because students, contrary to animals, possess a degree of consciousness that renders them at least partially immune to crude conditioning. For the sake of their mental health and by natural gift they resist the complete takeover of their will and actions by outside forces.

The "Problem" of Individualism

Unfortunately for the manipulators, there is always the "problem" of individualism, which is now well developed in our century—a natural possession of students in the higher grades who protest the system's destructive molding of their minds.

Not content with modern intellectualism, these young people are in search of something incredibly alien to our world picture: *a universal objective morality within themselves.* In their groping for a new world picture, the older students believe that love, freedom, peace, and the essentials of life come from within. But because this notion is contrary to all traditional views, their individualism is being challenged by social, religious, and educational institutions. And sadly and ironically enough, because all that schools have given them to work with is intellect itself, their tactics have involved little more than a shallow collectivism. So all their anti-war, anti-draft, anti–military-industrial complex protests have lacked human power because it has been drained away from the students by schooling.

So the educators "win" again. Students who rebel end up as powerless activists, dropouts, hippies, or members of other countercultures, seeking pseudo-meanings to life through drugs or other dangerous, empty pastimes. And those who don't resist? The "successes," those who are completely dominated by their intellect, are the most insidiously damaged in the depths of their psyches. They are the apparent successes in the competitive public and business worlds, each one out for himself, fiercely ambitious, clever, contemptuous of thoughtfulness and real concern. They measure and dispassionately count everything in sight, including the wounded and the dead, and are to all appearances the effective leaders who get things done in a single-minded, almost automatonlike manner.

They are the people who will use numbers and design complex systems to solve all human problems in the image of their world picture. But in human terms the problems still don't get solved. They are simply redefined in exclusively technological terms for quick solutions. And these purely outward "solutions," so typical of current society, are then passed on to the next generations through our institutions of learning.

These are just some stereotypes that are collective outcomes of our educational system. The personal and more intimate outcomes—the childhood that could have been but wasn't; the stunting of mental faculties; the daily fears, anxieties, pressures, humiliations; the heartbreak of helpless failure—are the private tragedy of the child who was robbed of his natural childhood, his mental health, and much that he could have become in adult years.

The Mechanical Approach to Children

The nineteenth-century mechanistic view of the world has expanded in modern days to include man himself. Our schools are caught up in this tragic concept, and our children now sense themselves as exchangeable and expendable human parts of a school mechanism:

> The main thing is not to take it personal, to understand that it's just a system and it treats you the same way it treats everybody else, like an engine or a machine or something mechanical. Our names get fed into it—*we* get fed into it—when we're five years old, and if we catch on and watch our step, it spits us out when we're 17 or 18. . . .[13]

Even those who declare themselves critics of our educational system view children as mere mechanisms. The noted writer on education Charles Silberman says:

> At each stage in development, that is to say—indeed, at each moment of time—the child has *some* mental apparatus, however primitive, that is the result of the interaction that has already occurred between the unfolding of his innate or "wired-in" mental structure and his experiences. And at each stage or moment of time, the child is extending that apparatus through probing and testing his environment—in infancy, exploring with his eyes, his mouth, his hands, his feet, his lungs; later on, through babbling, walking, talking,

playing, reading, etc. He not only stores information in his mental "files," he continually modifies and reconstitutes the filing system or mental apparatus through using it. . . . The sequence is not random, however; all children go through the same series of stages as, bit by bit, they construct their mental images of the world.[14]

One can almost hear the humming of the "wired-in" apparatus and the clatter of those files. One cannot resist the temptation to ask, "Is someone in the office?" It is once again business as usual at our schools as they methodically engineer the destruction of our children.

In a major effort of objective research, Patricia Minuchin of Temple University and her co-workers studied four schools ranging from the "traditional" and typical to the "modern," quite liberalized, child-oriented school. The study concludes that:

> In the final analysis, the impact of education does not lie so much in the tangible performance of the individual at any stage. *It lies, rather, in its effect on his continuing efforts to integrate experience into the ongoing processes of his own life and development.* (Italics added) [15]

It is indicative of our times that it was necessary to make a painstaking sociological study of a number of schools to arrive at this conclusion. Following the intellectual approach, human experience must be sought for by indirect *"research"* methods that by implication deny the validity of *direct* experience.

Intellect will kill any human observations made. Minuchin's study is replete with clarifying and helpful observations, but it is not in the nature of intellectual research to follow up findings with action on behalf of human life. That could only be done by people such as teachers who have *experienced* the situation, and only if individual experiences were considered *valid.* So the "scientifically" valid findings, devoid of personal experience, must remain powerless and are in effect being shelved everywhere among the welter of previous findings that are gathering dust. Consciousness alone could master the related meanings, appreciate the full weight of the crippling forces at work, and, fired by the feelings contained in experience, carry the findings into action.

A truth recognized but not experienced leaves us powerless to act upon it. It is this invalidation of human experience that preempts human solutions.

The Conditioning Farms

When one considers our educational system's emphasis on pure intellect at the expense of human development, it comes as no surprise to learn that the best-financed efforts in recent years at school "reform" have involved some kind of instructional technology.

The year that saw the inauguration of the "Educational Technology Decade" was 1965. It is difficult to appreciate the uncustomary excitement and extravagant claims with which electronics manufacturers, publishing companies, and government threw themselves into their various projects, never really making serious declarations about the benefits to children. Profit was the big motivation—not the children and the quality of their education. And even when educational development was a concern, it still had little to do with the expansion of children's minds or their human development.

L. Stolurow, director of the Computer-Aided Instruction Laboratory at Harvard, reflecting the view of many, would claim:

> Our present and most pressing problem is the lack of an empirically validated theory of teaching. In fact, we even lack a *useful* set of empirically validated principles of instruction that could form the basis for a theory of teaching. (Italics added) [16]

What Stolurow was saying is that the *engineers* still lack the educational principles useful for the development of machines that could deliver machine-regulated and controlled "teaching" rather than principles useful for *child-oriented teaching.*

As Anthony G. Oettinger of Harvard writes:

> Responses to requests like "describe a relationship," "define a concept," or "explain how something works" are well beyond the realm of current computer capability. Recognizing arbitrary English sentences by computer is still beyond the frontier of either linguistic or computer science.[17]

And Robert Glaser, director of the University of Pittsburgh's Learning Research and Development Center, clarifies for us the posture of intellectual science in relationship to the education of children:

> As a scientist, I am primarily concerned with the operational mechanism by which these goals are attained. Mechanism is indeed the right word; *it denotes the specificity required to carry out a reliable, replicable system.*[18]

But the techno-educators do try hard to appear human at times—at any rate, "efficiently" human. Professor Patrick Suppes of Stanford predicted in 1966 "that in a few more years millions of school children" would, through the computer, have a tutor like Aristotle.[19] Teaching machines would be called Plato III and Plato IV, and a great deal would be made of Individually Prescribed Instruction (IPI).

"Individually" means only that the student may cover the prescribed instruction at his own rate of speed. It does not permit "extraneous" goals or attempts to reach them in one's own way.

A programmed machine can provide information, but it is not capable of cultivating feelings or strengthening will, necessities for developing an open mental attitude that would later make possible flexible "integration of experiences." Living, breathing teachers are needed for this, not machines. With a machine a child will simply stare at information, play intellectual games with it, and memorize it to satisfy the preset program.

As Professor Lee J. Cronbach of Stanford has pointed out, computer-assisted instruction is a prescription for training and not for education. It is training *without* education, and it furthermore is the most primitive kind of training—the kind that can be realized only in behavioristic stimulus-response terms. It is, in fact, plain conditioning.

Skinner's rat in the box has now conjured up the Glaser child in the electronic cubicle. "We haven't thought much about what kind of citizens the school is turning out," Glaser told Silberman. "If we had started with that, we would still be designing the system."[20] A statement such as this calls for the most serious contemplation by anyone who still has doubts about the nature of science dominated by intellect. This reveals intellect's estrangement from man most explicitly—its basic mindlessness, its reliance on technology regardless of the human cost, and its general contempt for humanity.

The U.S. Office of Education is now widely disseminating the technological approach. Under the auspices of Research for Better Schools, Inc., which is in the Office of Education's Regional Laboratory in Philadelphia, the application of IPI has escalated from a single school started by Glaser to 23 schools in 1968–1969, to 169 schools in 1969–1970, with some thousand school districts reportedly applying for the project in 1970.

Government, the repository of public trust and tax funds, has quite obviously also failed to give much thought to the children's mental development or to consider the kind of students these schools may be creating. It is a crime against children, and it is a crime that is expected to involve eventually millions of children. The current estimate is that 75 percent of all children in all metropolitan areas will be involved by 1985—an ominous Orwellian deadline.

As destructive to the child's mind as they are, the worst current educational systems will look like quaint relics in comparison with what we shall someday see. Active intelligence, including intellect and consciousness, can never be programmed into a machine; nor can the cultivation of feelings, enthusiasm, and dedication to a self-chosen task be so programmed; nor can ability and powers of will unfold in a setting that is mechanically controlled. The future may not only see unused vital mental functions continually deteriorate; they may be actively encouraged to do so in order to conform with the severest of mechanical limitations.

Machines will then determine how human beings should develop.

Because of the demise of feelings and consciousness, unbridled drives are apt to flourish. The increasing use of technology in schools is but the most visible expression of spreading passivity in life. And passivity breeds unchecked drives that find an outlet in delinquency. Even now education is witnessing the proliferation of this delinquency at ever-earlier ages.

If automated instruction should come to prevail, we will bring on ourselves the era of anti-man just as we have already brought upon ourselves the intellectually inspired era of non-man.

The Roots of Antisocial Mass Disorders

Accomplishments of the human spirit such as those of Goethe, Spinoza, or Einstein could never have been wrung out of the substance of our current intellect-drenched educational system. Rather, they can only be realized in spite of it by resilient and larger personalities whose human spirit prevails, and whose self-chosen agony and sweat bestow on humanity the gifts to preserve its humanness.

Because of the formal schooling we have received for several generations, intellect now dominates our way of thinking and our life-style. It has become the *foremost mass neurosis* dominating all walks of life of Western man today. Externalization, self-alienation, psychic fragmentation and compartmentalization, automatic control, inhibition of feeling and impulses, denial of consciousness for anything that could cause conflict: these are the fundamental defenses of neurosis and the fundamental nature of intellect.

Because this neurosis of intellectualism has become institutionalized in our educational system, our schools are turning out passive, depersonalized individuals abounding in insecurities and hostilities. These are the students coming out of our schools—students whose neurotic, intellect-created hates, fears, and aggressions are being hurled at society.

Upon graduation, students have become human beings fully prepared to participate in the mental breakdown of the nation. For the sake of their sanity, our children can no longer afford the schooling they receive today.

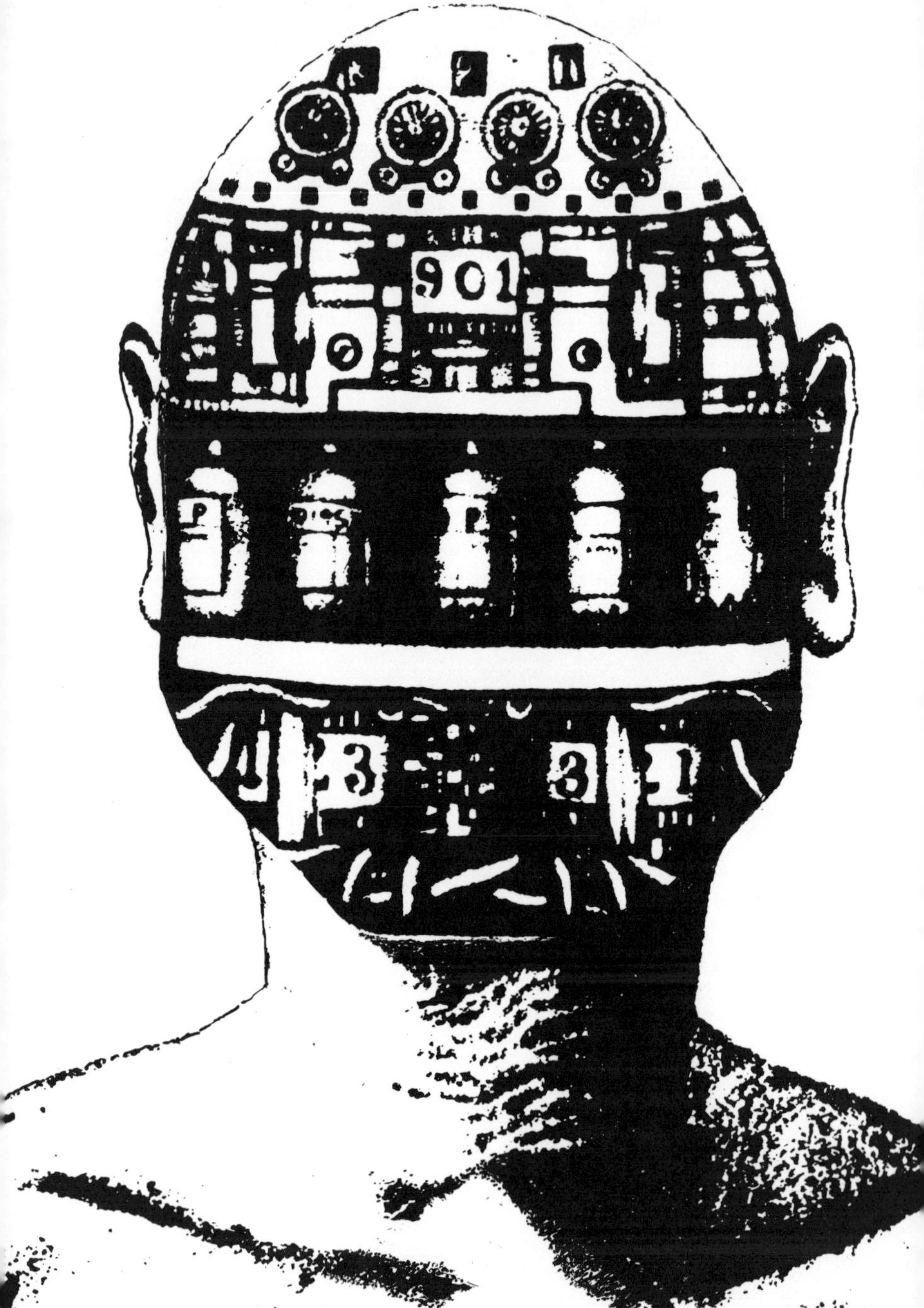
901

TECHNOLOGY: DESTRUCTIVE INTELLECT UNLEASHED

We all love technology. Gentle music and a discreet buzz will nudge us into awakening. We can glance at the latest news—flashed across thousands of miles—while dressing, turn on the orange juicer, fill the toaster with fortified, "factory-fresh" bread, and switch on the range for an instant coffee. Most of our homes are loaded with these latest conveniences. Life is just grand!

But do we really want orange juice every day, or is it a necessity spawned from owning that new automatic squeezer? And what do we really think of the taste of the technically reconstituted bread manufactured in the fully automatic bakery? Why do we accept eggs that have become increasingly tasteless—eggs laid not by hens pecking at nature in the backyard, but by those romanced with music, fancy lights, and hormones in order to speed up production? Why do we have to try Alka-Seltzer and like it after the instant coffee—or is the powdered milk the villain?

The answer to all these questions is that, quite simply, we have allowed technology to take over our lives. It determines where we live (available housing, accessibility to transportation), what kind of work we do (technology creates jobs), often our basic health (pollution), even our very thoughts (via the mass media). Technical necessities have indeed become our own necessities.

Our present machine-dominated society can easily be seen as the logical outgrowth of technological development, when one stops to consider that technology was never really *human*-oriented in the first place. Technology was, after all, a creation of our intellect. Just as intellect has grown dangerously out of proportion at the expense of all other mental faculties, so technology, its most visible reflection, has become frighteningly dominant over all departments of life, again at the expense of other human abilities.

The original idea behind technology was to make life *easier*—not necessarily better. Technological development has drifted since its beginning, advancing not so much to foster true human progress as to perpetuate itself, and the external way of doing things. This it has done, to the point that today technology no longer serves us; it is now we who are increasingly serving technology.

Technology is having disastrous mental effects, because all balance between technological necessities and human requirements has been lost. There is no human compensation, no rise to the challenge of proliferating mechanization, and no arousal of human ability and consciousness to secure a hold on technology. And there won't be, as long as we are fooled into thinking that technological progress is human progress.

So the scientific dream has become a mechanical nightmare. Descartes' utopian wish for a harmonious society has become the depersonalized assembly line, the polluted and materialistic havoc of the twentieth century. Henry Ford's hope for an easing of transportation problems has developed into congested highways and 50,000 traffic deaths per year in modern America. Biochemical research was the original idea, but poison gases somehow turned out to be the commoner result. We hoped for cheap and useful sources of energy; we also got the atomic bomb. And we found that military jets could be built through the same research that developed commercial planes. Clearly, the very depersonalized nature of technology ensures that the worst will usually result from any of its "scientific advances."

Technology not only dominates our world; its ultimate goal is the control of man himself.

The early technologists felt that although there would be necessities and constraints created by technology itself, man was still free in his inner life—free, in fact, to pursue at last that long-sought goal of happiness. As technology progressed, men were fascinated by the immediate results that could be obtained by setting standard devices in motion. Man, unfortunately, was *not* a standard device. But he could be far more effective if his spontaneous behavior were to be made deliberate and rational by preestablished *techniques.*

Using well-tested techniques, man's behavior could be fashioned into reliable and precise functions within organizations. These systems would be most effective if people or their behavior matched exactly and were easily exchangeable. In other words, if they were, in fact, *human machines.*

Choosing to ignore all that is human in man, technologists have experimented with precise systematization, division of labor, standards, production norms, and so on, in the never-ending search for the "one best way" to achieve the technical objective of human efficiency and not human goals.

If they ever succeed, they will have truly made technology our god, with man apparently fashioned in its image. When this happens, we really won't have to concern ourselves with the future of man. After all, machines can be replaced.

The World Trade Center and Other Defense Mechanisms

The last word in technology looms ominously over the lower part of Manhattan, New York City. It is called a building complex, but it is really a machine—the biggest machine in the world. It consists of two gigantic containers shipped in from the neverland of giants and erected to confound earthly micro-people with the new miracles of netherworld engineering. It is the World Trade Center.

To reach the World Trade Center one must ride over bumpy cobblestones past quaint nineteenth-century buildings with columns and gargoyles. The magnates of that time, while cruel and unpredictable, had not abandoned asymmetry, human dimensions, and human feelings. In contrast to these obviously human-made structures, the two immensely cold and massive towers of the World Trade Center invade the sky as the first generation of true machines inhabited by people who will be exchangeable parts in the organizations that assemble daily in a mechanically controlled, total environment.

Not only are men becoming mere parts of systems; the "best" systems in our technological society try to replace as many men as possible by cybernetics and place a single man at a central console to monitor the regulatory activities of the master computer, and react appropriately to anything that deviates from the programmed course.

In the World Trade Center, the mental activity of one man is all that is left (or needed) to monitor the computer's reaction to 6,500 remote sensors conveying information on pressure, water flow, humidity, temperature, power needs, and everything else that keeps the building "alive." The computer will automatically regulate all these systems, will kick in generators during brownouts or shut the entire system during weekends. The machine character of the building is physically apparent by its aluminum casing, its main support in the exterior walls, its intense internal heat that must be cooled by 100,000 gallons of water every minute, and uncounted technical devices that make it a self-regulatory mechanism.

What is the point of all this? Why was the World Trade Center built? Roger Starr, the executive director of New York's Citizens Housing and Planning Council, says, "The Trade Center is a vast condition of *ad hoc* arrangements." [1]

The reasons for the center's construction are still obscure. Not hidden, but just unclear to all. There was talk of an old railroad, a trade center proposal, the need for some state office space, the tax-exempt bonding power, or the desire of Austin J. Tobin, the Port Authority president, for a monument. Yet these all seem rationalizations for the unconscious, collective instincts of technicians.

In spite of criticism—mostly economic—and charges of inefficiency, the center was built in line with technology's obsessive motto:

> *If it can be done, it must be done.*

According to Glenn Collins, Richard G. Stein, a Manhattan architect, feels that there is great advantage in combining office space in aggregations. It is economically more efficient, and more advantageous organizationally, culturally(?), and "perhaps even humanly" (!):

> But at some point urban concentrations stop becoming efficient. Our studies on *energy utilization* suggest that for office buildings you reach a point of diminishing returns at about a million square feet.[2]

The World Trade Center has 9 million square feet of space.

There must be some forces in technology that go beyond rationality or efficiency; otherwise the center would never have been built. Says Jacques Ellul, an eminent writer on postindustrial society:

> For a long time it was believed that technique would yield a happy, harmonious society, a society in equilibrium, happy and without special problems. . . . The summum bonum was comfort. . . . It had been forgotten that technique means not comfort, but power.[3]

All the rational technological necessities foisted upon the hundred thousand people who now converge on the World Trade Center every day are not so rational after all. The technological rules, regulations, and necessities, such as traffic signs, are true necessities only *after* technology has become operative. They seem to provide an after-the-fact rational structure for the primary irrational intent of today's technology. Bigness and power, the compensatory defenses against deep-seated feelings of human irrelevance that are troubling technologists, are the real reasons for building such monsters.

The World Trade Center, despite all the glamour and pronouncements of progress, is really little more than a grand-scale metal manifestation of an entire society's neurotic defense.

The Mental Roots of Technology

The characteristics of technology will always betray their root in intellect. What the technologists try to pass off as efficiency, advancement, and the good of mankind is really only the scientific manifestation of our self-estranged intellect, that centuries-old neurosis which arose from the conflict between our unavoidably emerging individualism and our very fear of it. Intellect's answer to this conflict has always been to have us escape into the assurances of a purely external world. And what better way to do this than through the totally mechanistic, depersonalized route of technology?

If intellect is at the root of technology, drives are what are advancing it. Drives, those that emerge from our intellectually disowned will, dominate today's technology and encircle men in an increasingly illusory world. Those insecure, anxiety-ridden, power-hungry technologists who represent the rest of us are forever seeking new means to carelessly examined ends, always applying them immediately, no matter what shaky human purpose they might have or what they might destroy in the process.

Because our own drives are uncontrolled, *so is technology itself.* The only law it seems to follow is that of its own autonomous development. Raging on with utterly no interest other than in its own maniacal perpetuation, technology makes the very suggestion of a "technological humanism" an absurd impossibility. Our only hope is for a *humanized technology,* and this would require delving back into the roots of our *personal* problems in order to put man at the center of this world again. Only then may technology change and begin to work for man's good.

The Conflict

Technology presents man with a very human conflict. Starting in the nineteenth century with the Industrial Revolution, which lured rural inhabitants into the bursting slums, up to the present time when factory workers endure the assembly lines to get pay rates far exceeding those of some learned professions, technology's inherent economic control has forced men to make the choice between a personal failure or a "mass success."

As Jacques Ellul puts it:

> Only two possibilities are left to the individual: either he remains what he was, in which case he becomes more and more unadapted, neurotic and inefficient, loses his possibilities of subsistence, and is at last tossed on the social rubbish heap, whatever his talents may be; or he adapts himself to the new sociological organism, which becomes his world, and he becomes unable to live except in a mass society.[4]

There is no place for the individual in technology. Indeed, as Robert Jungk, a noted writer on behalf of the humanization of technology, says, "Considered from the modern technical view, man is a useless appendage."

Man is not only useless—his very humanness is a threat to a mechanical system that would run better without any personal interference. Technology wants to remove all human variability and originality, and it is beginning to do just that. In their thorough studies of technology, Lewis Mumford and Jacques Ellul have warned how the technicians' self-delusions are being cast like a net over the whole of social life. Says Ellul:

> True technique will know how to maintain the illusion of liberty, choice, and individuality . . . but . . . it will be inadmissible for any part of the individual not to be integrated in the drive toward technicization. . . . The individual will no longer be able, materially or spiritually, to disengage himself from society.[5]

The ideal of technical intellectualism is to have ultimately all perceptions pass directly to the brain without going through consciousness. This would ensure complete control, reliability, and maximum "productivity" of people. It is now done by operant conditioning, the new and burgeoning "behavior technology," but it may soon be possible by electronic means. Man would then come closer to what technology really wants of him: automatic response to it. When this happens, there will no longer be a conflict. There won't be anything human left in man.

Manipulation: The Modus Operandi of Technology

If the inherent power of technology does not stamp out our humanness, technology's manipulators will. They are presently manipulating our entire civilization.

Manipulation is inherent in any technique that bypasses consciousness. Because technology involves increasingly intricate complexities, it keeps most of us unconscious of what is happening, what we are doing, and why. We become depersonalized automatons, mere robots manipulated to keep the machinery running smoothly.

Because consciousness is the power of powers, in the face of it, all manipulation comes to a screeching halt. Not wanting man to be manipulated, Mumford and Ellul fear technology's promotion of progressive unconsciousness, while technophiles such as B. F. Skinner are exultant about the prospects of a world that is one giant machine controlled by the technology of behavior devised by a "cultural" designer.

The technologists' task is not simply to dim consciousness; the battle is also about *how* consciousness is used. The power of consciousness tends toward good if it is created out of the self, but subject to intellect it is perverted to the calculated manipulation of those who are less conscious. It is here that the manipulators step in.

Because machines have made work so monotonous for us, we get restless and inattentive on the job. We must be made to respond to our own drab tasks in the most polite and effective way possible.

One of the crudest ways to do this is in the pressure used in factories today that employ the self-arresting production line. Because production comes to a halt whenever a worker lags behind, the slacker feels guilty toward his fellow workers. Knowing his lagging is keeping them from earning their wages, he will resume the collective tempo in spite of distress or fatigue.

Physical fatigue has been mostly eliminated and mental fatigue is now the big problem. The depersonalized, rote nature of technical work has become the main source of discontent among restless, angry workers who resent the fact that they are not personally needed—that except for regulated spastic twitches required at the assembly line, they might as well be dead.

Because human discontent means bad business, a study of human behavior in industry is on the rise, and for only one purpose: technical efficiency.

According to McKeen Cattell, the founder of the Psychological Corporation:

> The development of technology as a science and its application to the control of human conduct . . . may in the course of the coming century be as significant for civilization as has been the industrial revolution.[6]

Many managers do not hesitate to admit that behind a public relations facade their psychologists and social scientists are management tools whose skills are used for human control. Cessna Aircraft and Atlantic Refining have furnished examples of management's practice of pressuring recalcitrant individuals into conformity with a "majority" by means of "group conferences." General Foods is convinced that "leadership" and persuasion would prove most effective in directing the thinking and conduct of its workers, while the Life Insurance Sales Bureau declares, "We need not change human nature; we need only to learn to control and use it." The Harwood Manufacturing Company and American Cyanamid both learned to lean heavily on group techniques to ensure management control. Motivation studies, selection devices, role-playing, sensitivity training, and especially counseling all proved to be helpful schemes to provide management with ever-subtler means of control.[7]

None of these programs has any pretense about really helping the worker. Management simply wants to manipulate the worker back to work. After all, the aim of technology is bigger and better business, not happier and healthier human beings.

Technologists are also manipulating man into consumerism. For the economic "good" of the country, planned obsolescence is required. We have become a throwaway society populated by throwaway people whom technologists have seduced into contemptuous use of the anonymous technical products that surround them.

Because our competitive industry has a built-in appetite for expansion regardless of need, what planned obsolescence cannot handle, advertising will. Advertising simply *creates* needs for us. So we buy useless products, all the while unconscious that we were manipulated into having to have them in the first place.

America the Technocracy

The biggest manipulators of all are often not technologists making plans for big business; they are the technocrats who are running our very society.

One has only to attend any New York City mayor's cabinet meeting, as this author did for years, to see technocracy in action.

An observation of the people attending one particular meeting all too clearly showed that the old-time professionals experienced in their fields had given way to the managers, systems men, and generalists who depend above all on statistics, systems analyses, and computer projections. The shift was plainly from human initiatives and responsibilities to the exclusive engagement of technology to provide necessary improvement in all areas of public life—including cleanliness, order, and crime and fire fighting.

All discussions limited themselves to better ways of doing things technologically. There was talk about installing tamper-proof telephones and fire alarms and rock-proof fire-fighting equipment. A computer projection of a certain drug-infested neighborhood was presented, showing the relentlessly growing impoverishment and crime despite the number of police on duty and community action, communication, or "systems."

When this author asked the people who made the projection to feed into the computer a hypothetical factor X representing an estimated possible mental improvement by "ideal" schooling, he was told that it was an impossible task for the machine. As a matter of fact, the computer people had never even considered pursuing this kind of burning human issue with their treasured technology.

Human issues are rarely considered anymore, government being most interested in how man can best be manipulated (not *helped*) by technology.

To attend this important meeting involving the plight of 8 million people was to see the old world view in full effect. The human suffering of a city plagued with all the greatest woes was regarded as a technical process that called only for programs, schedules, and timetables.

It was as if the city were empty of *people* except troublemakers requiring technical management. No humanness or initiative was attributed to the citizens; the only issue at hand was how best to control them.

And yet, for all their faith in the power of technology, people came stumbling out of the mayor's meeting arrogantly puzzled about the alarmingly troublesome behavior of the city's workers—the psychiatric conditions, alcoholism, drug abuse, absenteeism in body or mind, cost of disruptions, strikes, disorderly conduct, rising crime . . . what *was* causing all this irksome chaos that was impeding production? Why, even now, machines were wasting away, unused, unattended, and rusting amid the disruptive human turmoils. Something would have to be done about people . . . !

Electronic Hallucinogens

Nowhere is technology's strategic aggression against man as evident as in the mass media, technology's own master product. As is customary for all things technological, the media are presented everywhere as "progress" and as a main resource of our civilization. News reports, major events in politics or entertainment are today considered obligatory viewing. One is made to feel an outsider if one hasn't joined the 800 million people who watched the Munich Olympics.

But television doesn't merely "educate" us into insensitivity with the news, or bombard us with its mindless entertainment; in their perennial search for weaknesses on the human front, the technologists have found that they can actually bind us to the tube by flaunting on the screen the new aggression and *violence* encapsuled in the unconscious.

Now the media no longer provide mere entertainment; we also have the vicarious pleasures of enjoying our own secret drives—unpunished, as we passively identify with the violence we view.

Young children are known to accept the events on the screen as reality. They also tend to imitate what they see and do not sort out a meaning at their early age, trusting their parents that the meaning they do receive will be the right one.

Formal psychological tests prove that "violence on television leads children who watch it to be more violent in their behavior." A surgeon general's report of 1971 found that children exposed to violent television programs were more likely to hurt their peers and hurt them more intensely than were children of the same age who had been watching highly active but nonaggressive sports events.[8]

Psychologists have also reported that "repeated exposure to televised aggression leads children to accept what they see as a 'partial' guide for their own actions." [9] And a large body of research on observational learning by preschool children confirms that children learn aggressive behavior equally from real life and fantasy-cartoon models.[10]

In these cartoon models, characters are flattened, riddled by bullets, run through grinders, and often subjected to numerous devastating assaults in quick succession. That there is no apparent pain or injury only encourages the child to build a mental world where the most vicious violence is all in fun, and pain and sorrow are nonexistent—or in any case instantly relieved by a drug.

Television offers mere secondhand knowledge, pure indoctrination that denies the successive affirmation process of trial and error, or any activity on the part of the child. Studies have shown that toddlers sit motionless in front of television sets, their faces drained in totally passive submission. When interrupted from the hard-hitting events of the screen, they are startled—as if awakened from a dream. Dr. T. Berry Brazelton, a pediatrician from Cambridge, Massachusetts, says:

> The disintegration of ego mechanisms which one sees in [the child's] hypersensitivity, and in the screaming, thrashing, and disorganized hyperactivity which ensues after a period of television watching in most children is evidence of *the cost* of such a period. . . . At older ages the reinforcement for passivity, for allowing all activity to be produced *for him,* must have a powerful influence on the child's capacity to handle his own aggressive impulses.[11]

Television is a great teacher of passivity. This passivity also causes violence, being the unhealthy counterpart to aggression that also leads indirectly back to itself. When we have become so passive that problems, conflicts, or frustrations can no longer be handled by planned action but only by emotional explosions, our aggression erupts.

The child who is not yet submerged in our amoral world picture is horrified by the crimes he witnesses, but he also finds himself trying to identify. He is disturbed by the drives so mobilized within him. He comes to love what he hates seeing. He has now acquired a new conflict—the *television neurosis*—only one of the many technologically induced neuroses.

One of the latest assaults on the mental health of this nation's children is televised "educational" programs. The hugely acclaimed *Sesame Street,* for instance, sponsored by both government and industry, is "teaching" in a way that ignores the child and his healthy mental requirements and fully exploits the educational purpose of the program as a "bait" to make him a captive victim of the technological mentality at the tender age of three to six —which is for life.

Mental health principles requiring the active awakening of the child's curiosity and love of knowledge are ignored. Instead, small children are being bombarded, whipped, and hit between the eyes by oversized letters and figures that rush at them screechingly.

This rape of their trusting minds and the highly premature intellectualization wound children deeply without their even knowing. They may remember these signs as they do with other TV horrors, but their love for reading is ruined. It may be no coincidence that 48 percent of Manhattan's children, most of whom have been watching *Sesame Street,* are now behind at least one year in reading skills. Objections from various quarters are simply being ignored on the strength of technological power and popular ignorance. And copies of the program's malformed moppets are now widely sold "to fill the need" created by the program.

Sesame Street's technological indoctrinations are

even more insidious. A child is given "magic glasses" with which he then "sees" a ringing telephone, a horn-blowing car, a typewriter, or a man drilling the pavement. Moppets that leave the child in doubt as to whether he is dealing with people, animals, or monsters provide silly ideas he would never have thought of on his own, like blowing up a balloon with a fan.

He is supposed to learn from this, for instance, what "most" means, but since our moppet is a crime boss threatening the other moppet's life unless he gets "most carrots he can get," the lesson for the child is no longer what "most" means but the legitimacy of a threat to life in the adult world. The little girl who refrains from bursting the balloon and scaring her brother *only* because she does not want to be put to bed without dinner (a lovely thought in itself) is also a part of the morality of not getting caught—the early unconscious primer for juvenile delinquency.

Sesame Street is a program where three-year-olds learn that letters can walk and make machine noises; that Sam the robot is an insistently friendly neighbor; that to be famous you need a huge mouth and outstanding ears; and, finally, that Count von Count, who looks and acts like Mephistopheles and is apparently a representative of natural science, always counts everything, and, finding flowers harmful (another nice technological suggestion), he counts the sneezes too.

Above all, the hapless child learns that the knocking, hissing, screeching technological sounds of this subhuman, intellectually clever puppet world comprise the reality he is growing into, courtesy of the tragically accurate unconscious self-image projected by parents, industry, and government—all partners in our modern barbarism.

Sesame Street is one of the modern phenomena that

make it absolutely impossible for a child to grow up mentally healthy. It is one of our daily crimes against children.

Children begin to absorb the lessons of television before they can read or write. In a fundamental way, this medium now creates in preschoolers a self- and world-image of what they come to expect for themselves and others. These are, in fact, *the standards of civilized society*.

And they certainly have time to absorb these standards. Preschool children are now reported to spend almost two-thirds (64 percent) and older children from one-fourth to one-half of their waking time watching television. By the time a child reaches fourteen, he has watched the violent assault or destruction of nearly eighteen thousand human beings. As he graduates from high school, he will have spent twenty-two thousand hours in front of TV—twice as many as in school. And perhaps five thousand of these hours, nearly half of the hours in school, he will have spent watching commercials.[12]

Television has taken possession of *everybody's* waking time. It dictates what we see and hear for a cumulative average of ten years of our lifetime—with two of those spent watching commercials.

Why this craving for external pictures, instead of reading a book to enliven one's own imagination, or experiencing one's own life? Beyond television, why movies, photographs, posters, images everywhere? Why is every blank wall now soon emblazoned with glowing pictures?

Modern electronic images have passively replaced an inner imagery of thought that man has gradually lost since the Greek era. Greek literature shows that the Greeks thought in terms of vivid imagery, pictures that expressed their mental life. But our modern replacement is a dangerous one, for the Greek formed his *own* images; he formed reflections of his *own* perceptions. The ancient Greek would have considered the surrogate electronic imagery dangerous ghosts or demons that sought to enter into the shadows of his own soul; he would have thought it madness to abandon himself to external, unreal pictures or to live by their influence. To him such behavior would have been hallucinatory!

The technologists have found this deep human craving for lost imagery highly exploitable. While entertaining us, they have painstakingly researched the exact limits of human tolerance to advertising, the creating of needs for their products. That tolerance is rising, and so is advertising.

The huge success of reducing generations of people to abject mental passivity is materializing in the throngs lining up at movie houses, and in entire families sitting around a TV set daily for hours at a time. This passivity is now successfully subjecting people to the manipulative advertising of technologically invented needs. The implicit message is that the limitless consumption of technology's products is a necessity if you want to belong, to be loved, to be successful, healthy, young, democratic, and free.

Here technology reveals its true faceless inhumanity. It is not recognizable in what technologists think they are doing, in the glamour of technological achievements, or in the adult's seduction by its beckonings. It is in the heartbreak of seeing the pale faces of children abandoned to the electronic hallucinations that bring to their open and trusting minds precocious intellect, depersonalization, aggression, violence, indifference to suffering, cheap and degrading fantasies—all when they seek only humanity and self-assurance. It is in the destruction of their minds in their daily sessions of conditioning to all these specters that have become their reality, and the ensuing passivity as a mental style that prepares them to be the complying members of the technological age.

In these lost faces we can at last clearly read the big lie perpetuated through the unconscious of technologists. If we cannot, it is because we ourselves have become part of that lie. It is the sacrifice of concrete *men* to the technological model of abstract *man.* If we are insensitive and indifferent to or permissive of the child's media addiction, we are part of that lie—willful destroyers of our children's mental development.

Out of Control

Technology is out of control. This has happened because what is really out of control is that sector of our mind which places technology indiscriminately at the center of its existence as the external counterpart of its inner self-estranged compulsions. Technology is simply the reflection of our own inner intellect-based neurosis.

The most obvious sign of technology out of control is in our exploitation of nature. We see the effects of this self-destructive condition by looking out any window to mournfully observe the ugly, dirty, ravished, and disemboweled scenery that was once luscious, colorful nature ringing with life.

Technology out of control has also infiltrated the entire social structure. Economics, industrialization, and the problems of product surplus have led to the intentional building of a consumer society, a regressive, passive, neurotic society that is increasingly subject to mass exploitation through the false lures of more for less and something for nothing. And yet so self-estranged have we become that we often view this as human progress rather than the actual *exploitation* of man that it actually is.

More recently, and most ominously, applied intellect has taken hold of man himself. Technologists have now turned to the social masses, to concentrate on the human mind itself. Manipulatory reinforcement techniques in education and mass communications are enslaving man's dimmed consciousness in entirely new ways. And in all these chaotic instances, the virtually complete acceptance by our culture is the measure of our collective insane mental condition.

Unfortunately, most proposals expected to improve our mental and social woes are spawned from the same mentality that created the problem in the first place. They are technological solutions revolving around external manipulation, mind-altering drugs, psychotechnology, behavior technology, brain implants, psychosurgery, and so forth. These all belong in the category of mental self-mutilation. They are indeed evidence of a new, yet widely unrecognized advancing social psychosis. *When self-estrangement proceeds to self-mutilating practices among us, this constitutes genuinely psychotic behavior.*

So now our personal neurosis can be found duplicated in the broader social system. Our self-mutilating educational, scientific, and technological systems, parading always as "progress," really reflect our individual mental problems. In short, we now have *institutionalized insanity.*

The tremendous, uncontrolled power of technology makes our general psychotic condition even more frightening. The natural scientific model of viewing the world as matter and nothing else is indeed a culturally determining obsession; the technological approach based on this very obsession adds *action,* which will enable us to complete our mental breakdown.

It should be ominously clear that the hour of decision between men *or* technology is drawing near. Man as man cannot be absorbed into the ever more ponderous technological necessities without mental incapacitation and ultimate subhumanization. If we allow things to continue plunging ahead as they are now, man will one day find himself nothing more than a part of the vast technological machine that we are creating out of this universe. Then it will be too late to do anything about it.

Technology in itself is not an evil thing. It is merely a reflection of our own mass neuroses, taking whatever direction our self-estranged minds will have it take. If we were to put ourselves at the center of our world again, if we were to understand the necessity of positive individualism *and* the nature of intellect, we might still be able to tame the powerful ghost of technology.

We would reject much of our current technology and build another kind of technology altogether, one that would aid men for healthy human purposes in order to accomplish a truly progressive human culture.

But we need to remember that this change must begin within ourselves. Technology alone will never change the course of things, for by itself it is merely an external answer to external problems. We must begin to reach within ourselves for a reaffirmation of sovereignty over our mechanical universe, for this alone can produce presence, strength, harmony, love, accomplishment, and human advancement. Once we know again who we really are, we can then *use* technology to achieve ends for the betterment of mankind.

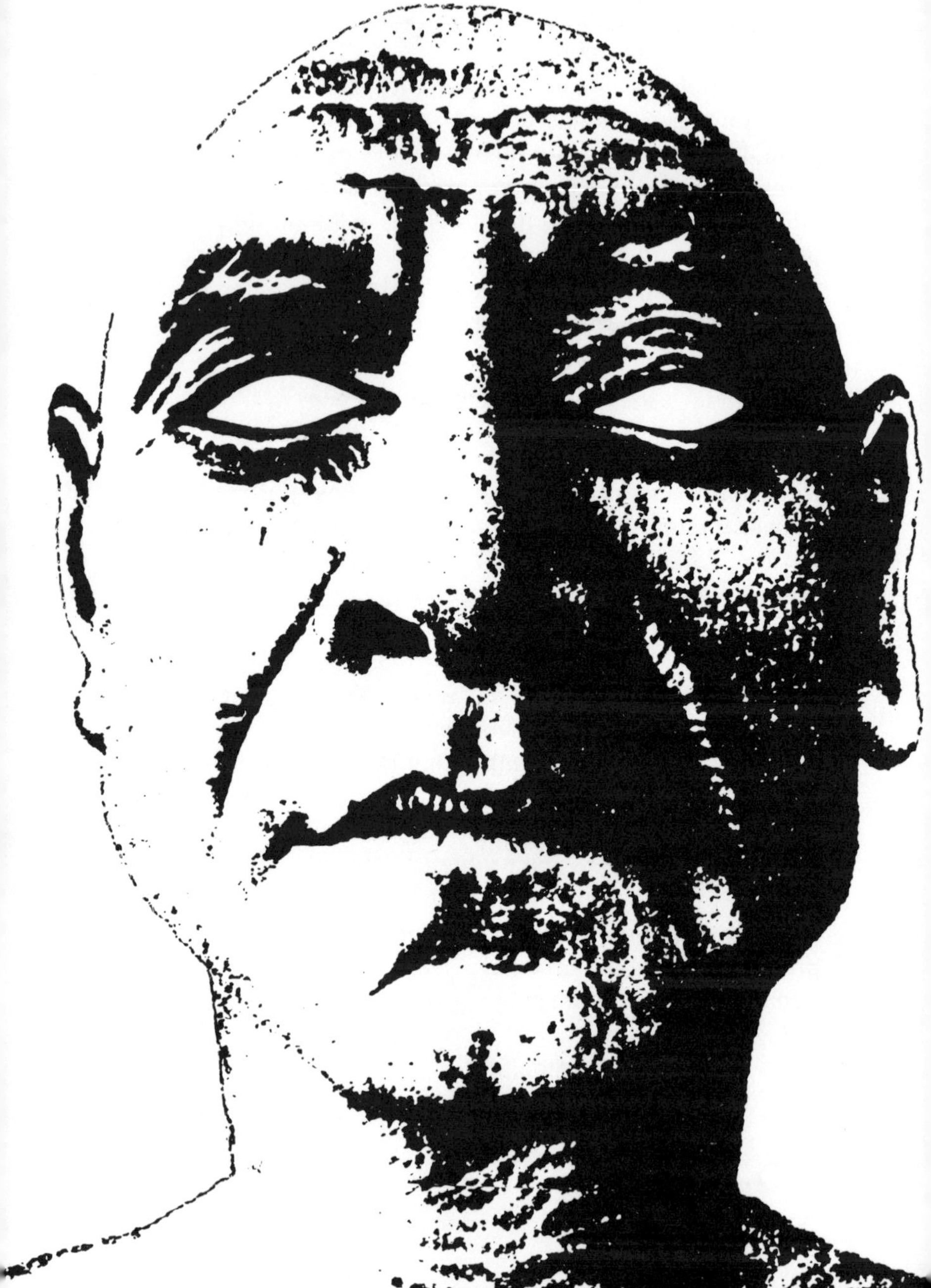

MAN'S CHANGING VIEW OF HIMSELF: HOW MAN'S HUMANITY WAS LOST

The reason why things are as they are in society today originated in the course of the history of billions of people who have walked the face of the earth. The thoughts, sentiments, ideologies, dogmata, truths, and beliefs of centuries past, supposedly long forgotten, rule our semiconscious life and form our present world picture. And of all the attitudes and beliefs that create our mental history, man's changing view of himself has played the most significant part in our lives. Time has bestowed upon us the gifts of intellect, individualism, and the potential of a new consciousness. But it has led to intellectual overgrowth, loss of feeling, will, and humanness—even mental breakdown. In a sense we are prisoners of the past, for our contemporary mental crisis is the sad consequence of a man-estranged view that has slowly evolved in the course of time. If we ever hope to get out of our present predicament, we must go back in time to see how we got here in the first place.

The Ancients

The history of mental development as it is most relevant to the present state of society begins in ancient Greece. Like the Egyptian before him, the early Greek's mind was immersed in mental imagery. His "thoughts" consisted of spontaneous images that made up his reality. What he pictured, he also felt and willed. Homer's epics (c. 800 B.C.) vividly demonstrate the rich imagery of which the Greeks were capable.

Daybreak, for instance, was never a mere sunrise, but the actual appearance of a goddess—rosy-fingered Dawn—who spread her arms to awaken the people. In this imagery, man did not place himself alongside nature as a separate being. He did not yet understand himself to be an individual human being, capable of personal joy, suffering, or achievement. Rather, he saw himself as an integral and unidentified part of the world around him, and thus he did not separate the experience of man from the experience of nature.

In time the Greek began to experience his first tentative concepts. A vague hint of abstraction was in the air, and the statement of Pherecydes of Syros (c. 600 B.C.) that the source of all being was the "good," which he then felt he had to give the name of a being (Arizon), clearly shows the conflict between the gradually fading imagery and the slowly emerging thought. A concept was replacing a picture in the Greek's mind.

The struggle between imagery and reason grew, the latter having gained relentlessly during the sixth and fifth centuries B.C. The historian Plutarch relates how servants of Pericles brought their master a one-horned ram they found in his pasture. The priest Lampon interpreted this to mean that Pericles would rule alone in a government usually ruled by councils, but Anaxagoras, cutting open the ram, showed that the *cause* of the deformity was a malformed brain and skull. Meaning and cause were now in competition as pictorial consciousness and conceptual intellect slowly began to separate in the Greek mind.

As reason began to free the Greek from the mental captivity of living pictures, there occurred a separation of the individual from nature and his fellowmen. A new mental freedom and individual dignity were born, and there was a sense of self-direction freed from the bondage of compelling divinities.

With this same separation from nature, however, man first came to feel *self-doubt* and estrangement. Confining as the fatalistic pictorial imagery had been, at least it gave man a way to experience himself as "real"—to perceive his own meaning in relation to the world at large. When he became conscious of himself as a separate being, man was suddenly torn away from all that had once defined the very meaning of his existence. He now had to justify himself and explain the world.

The Sophists acknowledged this mental detachment and actually played upon it. Protagoras said, "Man is the measure of all things, those existing, that they are, those nonexisting, that they are not." With personal thought now seen as sovereign, there was no need for an *objective* world view. Who cared what the world was really like, if man perceived it only in relation to himself and for himself? "Truth" was soon abandoned, replaced by the power of thought to *control* man's affairs.

The Sophists represented one of man's earliest abuses of freedom of thought. The effect of their misrepresentation of intellectual power as pure objectivity can still be seen today and has actually grown into a high art. A number of so-called scientific disciplines—sociology, psychology, psychotechnology, and behaviorism among them—are steeped in Sophism and would not exist without it.

A Highlight in the Development of Thought

The zenith of Greek thought came with Socrates, Plato, and Aristotle in the fifth century B.C. The tremendous mental steps taken by these philosophers were to have momentous significance for Western civilization.

Socrates felt that thoughts drawn in the right way from the innermost part of one's being reflected a world order, that is, thought unclouded by emotions could be objective thought. His student Plato was confident that this occurred in Socrates and could happen in all of mankind, and taking this a step further, Plato began to speak of the idea being reality itself—the true existence. Time and space became mere reflections of ideas, which took the form of matter as perceived by man.

Plato saw the soul divided into the areas of thinking, willing, and feeling, and he understood human progress to depend upon thought's command of the other two.

Plato's understanding of the soul represents a basic concept of mental health. When one of these *abilities* of thinking, willing, and feeling is impaired, or when they are in conflict with one another, mental disruption can be expected. Our own mental problems of today can be at least partially traced to the loss of the old Greek ideal of the integration of thought with feeling and will.

While Plato understood the thing itself to be only a shadow of the idea, which was the true reality, Aristotle saw the idea as only one aspect of reality—the aspect that the activity of thinking could lift out of the object. Matter itself, which could not be lifted out, was the other aspect of reality. Together they form the objective reality of man.

If the object observed was the soul itself and one submerged oneself into one's soul, one found the idea as the total reality, according to Aristotle's definition, for now it was both the subject and the object, an active and effective force superseding bodily forces. By this reasoning, Aristotle elevated the faculty of thought to a level of significance and importance never before approached. This accomplishment was the highpoint of a thousand years of development of thought in Greece.

Modern man can hardly comprehend Aristotle's concept of thought, an extraordinary inner mental activity sadly unrelated to our own contemporary instant, automatic intellectualism.

Thinking has now become a passive processing of facts rather than an actual process itself. The comprehensive understanding of thought as an ability that could be harmoniously united with feeling and will to provide man with a total experience was the highlight of thought in Greece.

Unfortunately, the unified concept of the soul was later lost. Plotinus (A.D. 205?–270) saw thinking no longer as a faculty that embraces the full life of the soul, but in fact as a screen that masks it. Conceiving any spiritual reality as *beyond* all thinking and only accessible to faculties that transcended thinking, he and his followers turned to mysticism, the approach to spiritual truths by way of feelings.

Greek thought had run its course. Thinking had lost its universality as a faculty combining feeling and will, and cold spineless *intellect* began rearing its head.

The Church and Man's Mind

As the centuries went by, thinking began to fade as an independent force altogether, being dominated by religious dogmata. Freedom of thought had no place within the Church, but in the face of advancing rationalism the Church saw the need to define man within a manageable scope.

In the ninth century A.D., the Ecumenical Council of Constantinople declared that man was divided into body and soul and the soul had only spiritual qualities. Man as a spiritual entity was abolished. To view man in a *human* way, to regard man as a spiritual entity of his own rather than as a mere function of the newly defined soul was actually considered heresy.

The result was that Western man was forcibly disowned of that which he had come to consider his innermost being. This humanless view of man of the first millenium A.D. has a tragic parallel in our times, for we have again tended to disregard him as a whole human being. Now man is described as little more than body, having only *psychological* qualities. Now the human aspect of his nature is ignored with equally disastrous results.

The established Church continued to widen the mental schism between belief and thought. The original message of Christ, "The truth shall make you free," had long been forgotten in the dogmatic division of sentiment and thought, of belief and knowledge. No longer conscious of "the world of ideas" cherished by earlier men, the Europeans were ready for the mental development already set in motion by the Islamic invasions of the eighth century A.D.

With the Church's consignment of the spiritual and supernatural to a strictly prescribed faith, man was left with little else to "think" about but the practical world. As a result, the European was highly susceptible to *Arab rationalism,* a form of thought that was totally materialistic. With the Arabs came new advances in mathematics, astronomy, medicine, and the infant natural sciences. So great was their influence that when the Arabs departed from Europe, a *depersonalized intellectualism* had become a force deeply embedded in the Western subconscious.

The Rise of Intellect and the Fall of Consciousness

The second millenium A.D. saw a burst of intellectual curiosity about the physical world never before known. A new interest awoke in mechanical energy, in communication, in the production of goods. The intellectual ability to combine the concepts of wind or water power, blade, wheel, and grinding stones led to mills and other crafts so typical of the Middle Ages. Print was introduced and navigational instruments invented, leading to a quickening of trade, communications, and discovery. The age of world discovery began, and the ships of Columbus, Vasco da Gama, and Magellan ventured into the open seas. In the fifth decade of the sixteenth century alone, in an historical and notable stark lightning flash of intellect, Nicholas Copernicus published his *De revolutionibus orbium coelestium,* Vesalius the *De humani corporis fabrica,* Geronimo Cardano a treatise on algebra, while Fracastoro announced the germ theory of disease. An increasing elite of new men were now ready to take a harder look at natural laws and the mechanics of things.

Galileo's Fateful Choice

This strictly physical interest in things was carried to an extreme by Galileo, as a result of his own ironically subjective analysis of man's senses.

> As soon as I form a conception of a material or corporeal substance, I simultaneously feel the necessity of conceiving that it has boundaries of some shape or other; that relatively to others it is great or small; that it is in this or that place, in this or that time; that it is in motion or at rest; that it touches or does not touch another body; that it is unique, rare, or common; nor can I by any act of imagination disjoin it from these qualities. But I do not find myself absolutely compelled to apprehend it as necessarily accompanied by such conditions as that it must be white or red, bitter or sweet, sonorous or silent, smelling sweetly or dis-

> agreeably; and if the senses had not pointed out these qualities, language and imagination alone could never have arrived at them. Therefore, I think that these senses, smells, colors, etc. with regard to the object in which they appear to reside are nothing more than mere names. These exist only in the sensitive body, for when the living creature is removed, all these qualities are carried off and annihilated. . . . I do not believe that there exists anything in external bodies for exciting tastes, smells, and sounds, etc. except size, shape, quantity, and motion.[1]

In this statement Galileo differentiated between "valid" and "invalid" sensory perceptions, breaking down all objects perceived into "real" and "illusory" qualities.

Valid were those with *physical* attributes: size, shape, quantity, and motion; invalid were those *experiential* senses of color, taste, smell, and sound. (Sound was only later relegated to the valid category, having been broken down into measurable wave frequencies and amplitude.) In short, if it could be measured, it was real; if it could only be perceived, it was not. Galileo's followers were so blindly infatuated with his division of real and illusory qualities that they gave his theory the status of objective law!

Galileo's "law" made man's general consciousness —the complete, human experience of things—of little importance. Depersonalized intellect now reigned supreme even over experience, and the humanly valuable *and* truly valid ingredients of consciousness, such as imagination, intuition, and inspiration, now counted for nothing. Only that which could be grasped strictly by intellect was declared to have any reality.

This quest for cold factual knowledge that totally ignored the human element clearly showed the obsessive nature of intellect. And soon man would compound his error by assuming that this mechanical, measuring approach to natural science could be applied to everything else in life—including *himself.* A new "objective" view of man was emerging on the historical scene, and it would have disastrous consequences in the centuries to come, even up to our own time.

The New Society

If Galileo applied Nominalism—the view that what is not physical is mere words—to natural laws, Descartes applied it to man himself and to his society. Recognizing man as a creature with strong personal drives, Descartes proposed an absolute, authoritarian political system that he thought could control man in the same way that natural laws "control" natural science.

This suggested system was a blueprint for the mechanization of people, not yet by machines, but by autocratic authority, order, and regimentation. Men had become exchangeable "parts" within the social organization.

Individualism had no place in a society where man was defined by how he functioned within the system. However expedient in "running" our world this collective view of man must have seemed, it left little room for responsive, inner, human development.

Descartes expanded this exclusively external approach to man far beyond the political arena:

> If any means can ever be found to render men wise and more ingenious than hitherto . . . it is in medicine that they must be sought for.[2]

In this statement Descartes showed himself to be the precursor of an idea now promoted in our own time by scientists, the drug industry, and much of the new generation: the use of external agents instead of the development of inner potentials to find man's ideal existence. Sir Francis Bacon would carry this external approach even a step further with his interest in industrial exploitation.

The Dream of Francis Bacon: Technology

With extraordinary insight into the nature of the emerging sciences, Francis Bacon explored the possibilities of "effecting all things possible" through technics. And he made it rather explicit that by this he meant riches and material abundance.

Bacon believed that "knowledge is power," and by this he did not mean "consciousness is inner power" but rather that "intellect provides external resources." To achieve global expansion, he first suggested corporate organizations, operational systems, government aid, and division of labor in scientific technological work for the sake of efficiency, economy, and expeditious expansion. These proved to be important junctures in the mental development of Western civilization, for they would later herald the dehumanization of technological man.

Intellectual man had come to view the mathematical system of the universe as the total substance of reality. But man himself is not a machine, and mathematical certainties are not human certainties. This intellectual disregard of the crucial elements of man's mind—his consciousness, his feelings, his intuition, his will—was an invalid and dangerous assumption. This dehumanized view of mankind had set the stage for Western man's gradual mental disintegration.

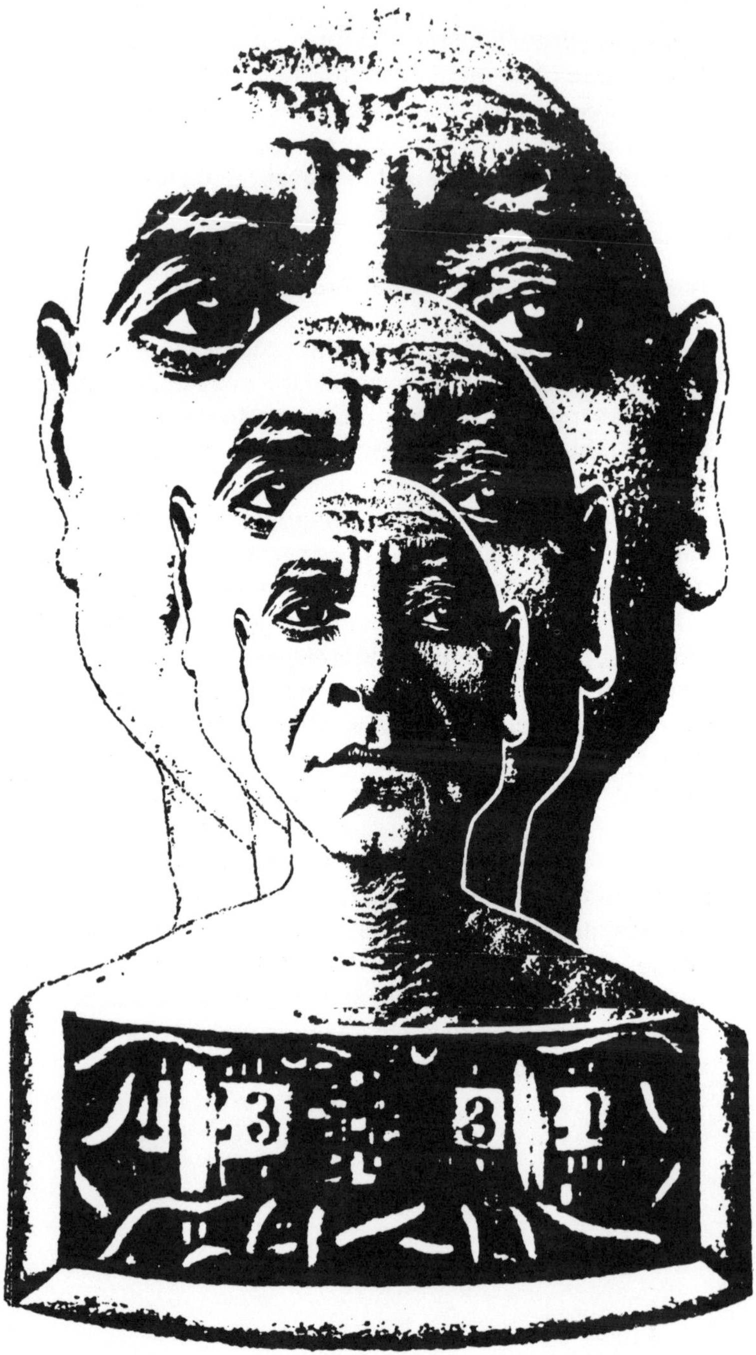

MODERN PSYCHOLOGY AND THE LOSS OF REALITY

The development of such human sciences as evolutionary theory, genetics, biology, medicine, psychology, behaviorism, and psychiatry has had much to do with man's present view of himself as somehow unreal and secondary to natural processes. Modeled after the natural sciences, these fields have tried to define man "scientifically"—to extract principles of life, mind, and man's purpose of being as they would natural laws. This so-called scientific approach to man has had the most dire mental effects. And of all the human sciences, none has had a more devastating effect on our self-image than the two main schools of psychological thinking that emerged at the beginning of this century. They are psychoanalytical psychology and behaviorism.

The World of Psychoanalysis

The psychoanalytical psychology created by Sigmund Freud was undeniably one of the most incisive developments in the field in this century. Its popularization of sexual drives, its probing of the unconscious, and its declaration of inaccessible depths in man that control his mind both shocked and fascinated the generally constrained Western world. Penetrating the horrendous and absorbing depths of a society conditioned by intellect, Freud set the previously purely descriptive field on a new inward course, one that legitimatized drives in general and the libido in particular as human "propellants," opening seemingly endless possibilities of self-discovery.

Earlier in the century the behaviorist John Broadus Watson had made the somewhat defensive statement that "no one has ever touched a soul, or seen one in a test-tube. . . ." [1] Now psychoanalytical psychology gave man a way to discover the nature and meaning of mental functions. Now "inner" action was plausibly and explicitly described, spiced with the sexual connotations of mysterious events: defenses, repression, regression, sublimation, and so on.

Here at last were activities of man's own doing. In a man-estranged intellectual society, this recognition of a person's inner reality seemed almost too good to be true. It was.

As a neuropathologist and natural scientist, Freud faithfully adhered to the accepted scientific criteria of what constituted reality. Flatly stating that the pursuit of psychodynamics was justified *until* the physical-organic causes of mental disturbances could be discovered (he also introduced the natural scientific model of thought in his conceptualization of psychodynamics as ultimately subject to physical-chemical dynamics), he further demonstrated the day's obsession with the physical sciences and technology in the *language* he used to express his ideas.

Repression, defense, and sublimation became "mechanisms"; the unconscious became unconscious "material." Regression could not possibly have been called an exotic name such as "disevolvement" or any other term having a purer psychic or living connotation; it had to relate to time, space, or movement. And the "soul" itself, a word totally unacceptable in a scientific age, became known as "psychic apparatus."

Freud's ideas themselves were concepts carefully construed to fit an intellectual age. Clearly, a mechanistic world had inspired the conceptualization of the id (drives), the ego (mediator), and the superego (social censor), the pillars—or should we say the conveyor belts—of psychoanalytic psychology.

Psychoanalytic psychology recognizes no inner reality of the individual. This is first obvious in Freud's conception of the id, which he sees as a certain sum of energy —lawless, valueless, and basically amoral—that forces its way from bodily needs to mental expression. Residing in the unconscious and thus being far removed from external reality (the *only* reality recognized by Freud), the id is actually defined as little more than a theoretical abstraction emptied of all *human* reality.

The ego is also denied a true reality. Defined as a mediator between the unreal individual and the real world, whose prime function is perception of world reality and adaptation to it, subject to the individual's *physical* maturation, the ego is actually conceived as formed by the world, which acts upon the organism. Here again thinking, feeling, and will are denied a reality, for they are seen only as a responsive *function* to the outside world, the only true reality.

The superego equally lacks ownership. Viewed as a mere *reflection* of the values, morality, and conscience that supposedly emanate from society rather than within individuals, it further denies man's own contribution to reality.

Probably the only human element in psychoanalysis is the actual give and take between therapist and client. It is certainly not in the theoretical frame of reference, where the eclipse of the reality of psychic events, the negation of human initiative, and the theme of response only move the old scientific-technological approach to a new setting—*inside* of man. The id, superego, and ego are veritable ghosts in this "psychic apparatus." They suggest the analogy of hot steam (id), the movement-confining block (superego), and the mediating lubricator (ego). They are simply a new expression of that great mental fixation of the nineteenth century, the mechanistic world picture.

Enter Behaviorism

Animals and slaves were once trained only in circuses or for the benefit of their masters. Ivan Pavlov changed all this with the scientifically established concept of conditioning, the precursor to the "reinforcement" now used by behaviorism.

Behavioral science made its first notable appearance shortly before World War I through John Broadus Watson. Evolving into a neobehaviorist system of "scientific psychology" through Clark Hull and B. F. Skinner, and others leading in the field, it gained pervasive influence over the teaching of psychology at almost every institution of higher learning in this country. And in its claim to be the last "scientific" word about man and all human affairs, it has also determined the approaches of other life sciences such as education, sociology, clinical psychology, psychiatry, philosophy, ethics, and political science.

In what appears to have been a reaction to the excessive "introspectionism" of German psychoanalytic psychology, the behaviorist set out to apply the classic tenets of physical science—measurability, predictability, and so on—having as a goal the measuring of behavior by quantitative methods (mass) and the control of behavior by manipulation of stimuli (motion). There was to be no room for "intangibles" and "unapproachables."

According to Watson, the behaviorist was to exclude "from his scientific vocabulary all subjective terms such as sensation, perception, image, desire, purpose, and even thinking and emotion as they were subjectively defined." [2]

B. F. Skinner has recently taken behaviorism a step further and defined all that is human as a mere by-product of the external world. Thoughts, feelings, memories, and values are all considered illusory and invalid—and useless in providing personal and social happiness.

With the old "unreal" explanations of man replaced by "scientific analysis," the behaviorist declares that external contingencies, once kept haphazard and chaotic by the idiotic self-illusions of "autonomous man"—thereby having conjured up all our social disasters—can now be brought into an external order. At last, having demystified the illusion of freedom and dignity falsely accepted by society for so long, a new nonautonomous man can soon emerge who is nothing in himself but "everything" as a useful part of an all-controlling system.

As with Descartes, the issue is once again not the advancement of man and his inner attributes, which would benefit society as a sum of *individuals,* but the foundation of a social system. And the behaviorist supports all this in the name of *science*—scientific analysis supposedly fighting the "prejudiced" opinions expounded by those ignorant ones who still delude themselves with their beliefs in man's thoughts, feelings, will, and consciousness.

Fighting behaviorism on the grounds that it is "trivial," "distasteful," "terrifying," or "leading to a kind of hell" is dismissed as a subjective argument that blindly overlooks the authority, power, and most of all the "proof" of "scientific analysis" and "experimental methodology."

Science has indeed become the religion of the twentieth century. And today's doubters are put to shame just as much as heretics ever were in biblical times. But we had better look carefully at what science is really doing, for in behavioral psychology alone, there are problems of theory, of fact, of application, of interpretation, of conclusion, of emotional bias, and even of self-deception that could lead us to a worse hell than early superstitious man could have ever imagined.

Man as Rat

Because of the overwhelmingly complex nature of the human being, simpler organisms were chosen for the behaviorist's experiments. And although the equation of man with the pecking pigeon or the bar-pressing rat is not particularly publicized, it is implicit in the writings of Watson, Skinner, Clark Hull, and, in fact, *all* behaviorists. Differentiating man from animal quantitatively and not qualitatively (the word "quality" is banned from the behaviorist's vocabulary, anyway), mental activities of the human being are actually derived from the performances of lower animals caged in Skinnerian boxes.

Behaviorism actually denies the psychological features of both man *and* rat. It studies one mental process only: the ability to be conditioned, which means to respond instinctively according to deeply ingrained survival mechanisms. This hardly encompasses the whole man—or whole rat, for that matter.

One behaviorist contention is that thinking is "behaving which automatically affects the behavior and is reinforcing because it does so" (Skinner, *Science and Behavior*). This concentration on external facts, or "whats," to the exclusion of meanings, or "whys," has resulted in such limited and ridiculous definitions of human events as cited below:

> A smile is an occasion upon which social approach will meet with approval. A frown is an occasion upon which the same approach will not meet with approval. Insofar as this is generally true, approach comes to depend to some extent upon the facial expression of the person approached. We use this fact when by smiling or frowning we control to some extent the be-

havior of those approaching us. . . . The stimulus comes to be effective in increasing the probability of that behavior and is produced by the speaker because it does so. (Skinner, *Science and Behavior*.)

Behaviorist literature is replete with such vapid pronouncements that describe an intellect that is broken up into conceptual bits that are no longer reflections of demonstrable realities. In reality, a smile at the wrong occasion with the wrong people present could cause precisely the opposite effect (try smiling when someone slips and falls to the ground), and a frown on other occasions could provoke hilarious effects, depending upon human circumstances.

The key experimental procedure on which most of the conclusions about human behavior are based is called "operant conditioning." What this basically means is that a rat learns that a pellet ("reinforcer") will appear when he presses the bar ("emits an operant response"). But the words "emit" and "operant" seem to acknowledge the rat's *initiative,* and this contradicts the behaviorist's theory of totally passive response. Recognizing the nonpassive, internal initiative implied in the stimulus-response theory, Skinner turned to the purely external "reinforcement of contingencies" postulation, thereby excluding all unmeasurable elements from man, rat, or psychology.

In other words, *the measurable became the only reality solely by virtue of its measurability.* Translated into life, this "truth" means that organisms, including the organism known as man, are completely controlled by their environment. This is the "truth" that now dominates our world picture.

Meanwhile, the pigeons and the rats continue to

apply their *whole* psychology. The rat uses his initiatives and ingenuity to obtain as many pellets as he wants, thereby preserving his ratness, while man, in accepting the idea that he is responding to the "dispenser mechanism" of environment and society, is now taking it for granted that these are the determining factors of his life. So a rat, incapable of absorbing great materialistic-mechanistic inspirations and indoctrinations and being oblivious to intellect, retains his wholeness as a rat—but man inevitably loses his wholeness as a man.

Deception as a Science

Animals can be conditioned on schedule because they have no understanding of themselves. But where the behaviorist can easily work *with* an animal's instinctual responses, he must work *against* man's consciousness, for people can only be conditioned to the extent that *they are unaware of it.* It is no accident that the behaviorist claims the most visible "success" with children, the retarded, and the mentally ill, for they are the least aware of any of us.

All of us are unaware to a certain extent, for life is permeated with subliminal situations, intentional or unintentional, by association or reward, that shape a personality when they are mostly or completely unconscious. There are immense opportunities for conditioning from birth, into preschool, school, military service, vocation, profession—in short, in all times and places of environmental influence. The less conditioning is noticed, the more powerful it will be. The entire struggle toward inner freedom consists in the shedding of these forgotten influences.

Consciousness tends to give man autonomy. This is not what the behaviorist wants:

> What is being abolished is autonomous man . . . his abolition has been long overdue. . . . Presumably, there is an optimal state . . . in which everyone is maximally reinforced. . . . Only by dispossessing him can we turn to the *real* causes of human behavior. Only then can we turn from the inferred to the observed, from the miraculous to the natural, from the inaccessible to the manipulable. . . . To man *qua* man we readily say good riddance.[3]

This is the language of behaviorism. And it is frightening talk, for it clearly indicates the behaviorist's unforgivable intent: to be the designer of a new race that would become increasingly responsive, but decreasingly conscious of being designed, until *man reaches a level of unconsciousness comparable with nature.*

And the work has already begun. Whoever reads *Beyond Freedom and Dignity* should be wary of the uncounted subliminal messages he is absorbing to this end. For example, on a single page (page 203), you're advised as follows:

> All that you can find in history is behavior
> machines make you more human
> teachers are worse than teaching machines
> initiatives deprive you
> the role of autonomous man to give human
> behavior direction has passed. . . .

These are just a few of the indoctrinations that are passed off as scientific laws by the behaviorist.

Despite the unfavorable book reviews, the angry attacks, and even the ridicule, behaviorism is not likely to be stopped. It is too much a part of our "scientific" age—too much the product of our man-estranged world picture that counts human beings as little more than parts of a larger system. Like its sister, psychoanalytic psychology, behaviorism views reality as coming from *outside* man, and it views his mental functions as mere response to this external reality. Both fields have mistakenly shaped their ideas from natural science, for by different routes they have devalued man to the point where he has no more meaning than nature itself. Human meaning has tragically become little more than a consequence of mass and movement in space and time.

Man as Man

There were a few isolated investigators of extraordinary resilience within our prevalent world picture who cherished the concept of transcendence. They had a loyal but, unfortunately, small following. Carl Jung's insistence upon the role of purpose in human development did not endear him to the spirit of the time. Nor did Alfred Adler fare much better with his emphasis on human goals as a powerful factor in personal mental health. Especially galling was his call for social interest when the world view was demanding social adjustment. And the prominent psychiatrist Karen Horney weakened her claim to broad acceptance in the world of psychology by embarking on another taboo of intellect: the concept of the "innate striving for self-realization."

The existential view of man as a unique being in the world and the seeking of optimal self-development remained at the fringes of official psychology. Frankl's existential "logotherapy," which sought to evoke in man a "will to meaning" that would be specific and personal for each individual, was completely ignored. And relatively few have even heard of gestalt psychology, with its heretical world view of seeing the meaning of parts as largely determined by their relation to the whole. Nor are its therapeutic techniques widely used, for they attempt to help the patient achieve self-actualization, to *re-own* the estranged, fragmented parts of his personality, to become "real," to develop the central core of his person.

But meanings do not enter into the current world view, nor are human meanings part of the mainstream of our official psychologies.

Behaviorism has had rats pressing bars for sixty years now, and with hardly a meaningful psychological insight of benefit to *man.* Rats may still find the vindication of their torture in seeing increasing masses of people pressing bars, buttons, and levers, courtesy of the same mechanistic obsession now enacted in social life.

Psychoanalytic analysis could offer much that is true and humanly helpful if stripped of its materialistic, mechanistic verbiage and attitude. In contrast, behaviorism, in its radical purge of man himself, will liquidate man, for it ignores his mind and closes the doors to any further mental development.

To place man in chains is now justified by nothing more than the claim that it is scientific to do so. In fact, the ultimate scientific feat will be accomplished when man joyfully embraces his mental slavery.

When intellect takes control and proceeds to order individual life, society, or an entire culture, man's mental abilities will be suppressed and ultimately destroyed. In the early years of this century Carl Jung gave warning of what was possibly to come:

> Sooner or later—in accordance with outer circumstances and inner gifts—*the forms* of life *repressed*

> (i.e., feeling, consciousness, intuition, etc.) *by the intellectual attitude* become indirectly perceptible through *a gradual disturbance of the conscious conduct of life.* Whenever disturbances of this kind reach a definite intensity, one speaks of a neurosis. (Italics added) [4]

This "gradual disturbance of the conscious conduct of life" has reached a self-destructive intensity in the 1970s. Its calamities and sorrows are boundless, and the fearsome gravity of the condition is revealed by man, who, after having gradually lost so much of himself, has now also lost his will to care.

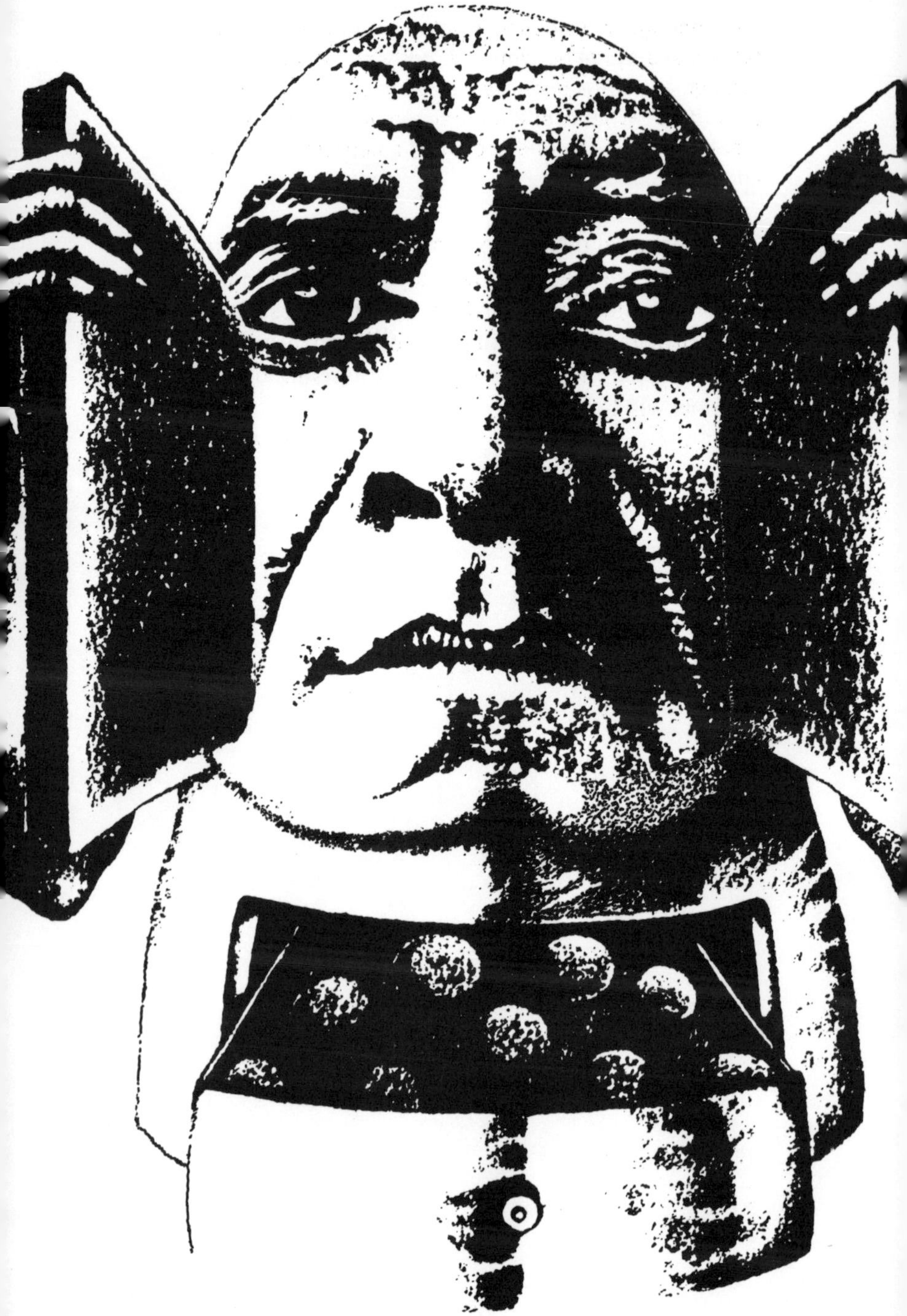

MENTAL HEALTH OF THE FUTURE

Modern man has had a mental breakdown. Robbed of his essential human substance, he has become neuroticized by intellect and rendered psychotically self-destructive by technology. If he is to avoid total annihilation, he must abandon his depersonalized, old world view and realize that ultimately his mental health depends upon a new world view that leads to a complete reaffirmation of man as an experience from within. In short, he must repossess himself as a human being. This means reactivating his thinking power, opening his mind, deepening his feelings, empowering his will, and, above all, turning back to the experience of intrinsic personal validity, the key to mental health.

It will not be an easy task. Generation after generation down the centuries has been gradually conditioned into viewing the world one single way, and that single vision had become stringently exclusive of any other way of seeing. If man is truly to build a new human world view, he first must *deview* the old. This means that he must become aware of his conscious and subconscious views of the world as long-conditioned states of mind. He must recognize those clearly cruel and dehumanizing actions he carries out based on such conditionings that put people through the relentless and crippling educational, scientific, technological, and economic stresses that are the invention of an inhuman society.

When he has finished deviewing, man must strive to form new views that reflect not only intellect, but also the overriding consciousness of whole man and his meaning in the world. The task will be difficult, for in the course of long mental neglect man has lost a great deal of his ability to become conscious, to really feel or even act beyond a conditioned state of mind. He must work toward a mental reconstitution—the systematic development of those mental faculties that had been lying fallow, distorted, misused, and sickened for generations.

Man must allow his mind to come alive again. His consciousness, feeling, and will must be liberated to rejoin and invigorate the long-neglected and rejected self. Man must begin his most urgent, supreme human liberation. This chapter will offer suggested ways to deview the old world picture and rebuild a new one in order that man may once again restore himself to full humanness for a mentally healthy world.

Deviewing the World View

Our intellectual approach to life has us believing that a point of view is invalid unless it is "objective." This must mean, then, that all human experience is invalid, for it is "scientifically" unmeasurable. Yet we must also realize that even within intellect there is no objectivity but only a consensus, because of the relativity of our senses and our limitations to strictly physical references on a conceptual level. Objectivity then, while unattainable in the physical world, is completely out of place in the mental world, for what counts there is reality. Experience, for instance, has no relationship to objectivity—only to reality. The feelings that are always part of experience are valid to us regardless of the object. We must learn to accept that *what we feel is indeed real.* Telling someone to be objective about something is really the same as telling him to ignore reality in favor of abstraction!

During the course of history, our infatuation with intellect allowed us to lose our "self-consciousness"—that acceptance of our own being as having a reality of its own within the larger universe. When early man's conceptualization separated him from nature, thus making him an individual entity, he felt anxiety in his new state of removal from the real world. He therefore turned his mind to physical, tangible things to support a new, totally intellectual reality. But this new, overintellectualized world cut man out completely other than as a physical being. If we are to deview the world around us, we must be conscious of our whole selves again. We must recognize our thoughts, feelings, and will as important and valid realities. These mental abilities that our intellectual world has ignored must be brought back into our lives—into every aspect, from the very specific areas such as education and technology, to general views about our societal behavior and our methods of modern research, on into that most precious area of all: *our very selves.* We must be conscious of our own essential being if we are ever to deview our old depersonalized world picture and create a new, human world view that will restore our mental health and make us whole again.

Deviewing Education

The most tragic and criminal consequence of our present world picture is our unchanging way of educating our young. It is in our schools that our future citizens are indoctrinated in the intellectual method, that narrow way of thinking that is destroying our society. In deviewing education, we must no longer view children as things to be molded. Nor can we continue to view intellect as the most important part of a child's mind.

Our education must awaken children to what they come to sense as their very own purpose in life. It must warm and deepen their feelings and enlighten, but not mold, their thinking. We must impart the skills and knowledge a child needs in a way that allows him to become *his very own and his very best,* whatever that may turn out to be. It is the school that must strike a chord in his human nature. It can be done by adhering to these well-tested avenues of true, natural learning: through imitation as a small child, through authority as a preadolescent, and through reason during the teens.

Naturally, this can be done only by teachers who have deeply experienced their own inner reality. Having achieved this mental level, they are likely to be disposed to do the right things spontaneously. Their concerns, approaches, and emphases will then flow from their basic human attitudes.

Deviewing Technology

Because its primary and *only* goal is to create an "expanding economy," technology has us working to obtain what we *don't* need; submitting to relentless conditioning to what we are told we need; and being constantly incited to consume extravagantly to keep excess production going. Technological necessities have become millstones that grind what is human in us to dust.

There is no *personal* benefit to any man in this purposeless, monotonous, mechanical "business as usual" world. The argument that workers must take industrial jobs because they can't support themselves in any other way is a hollow one, because it is our very own technology that has all but eradicated other possibilities. Nor can we argue that we need machines because they provide us with free time for doing more human things, for the time we spend working with these machines disables us mentally. Working with machines makes our wills superfluous; we then proceed to spend our leisure time passively, utterly dependent on the products we build, thus disabling our wills even further.

In deviewing technology, we must ask ourselves what *human* benefits exist; all that is simply technology advancing technology for technology's sake must be eliminated.

Deviewing our "Scientific" Method of Research

Instead of expanding man's mind and knowledge, our method of research is, ironically, a *limiting* process. It constitutes a sequence of closing mental doors.

The first limitation was the official acceptance by science of size, shape, quantity, and motion as the only reality. This closed our mental doors to the remaining universe. Then this materialistic science needed *methods* of viewing the material world, and further doors were closed to aspects of matter not accessible to *preordained* methods. These scientific methods became operational in technology, and technology's own necessities closed the doors to scientific methods that would not further technological ends. Finally, technology itself became fully subject to economics, which then closed all of its doors to any technology that would not serve economics.

Men now understand the crudest laws of mass and motion, but few understand true scientific methods. Even fewer understand the laws governing technology, and no one understands the laws of economics. These are all mental doors slammed in our face. We should open our minds to think about *all* aspects of a subject, regardless of its particular "usefulness."

Deviewing our Negative Self-Image

The film *A Clockwork Orange* portrayed in gory detail the ultimate result of a dehumanized world view. Here man was lost to man, as unfeeling, passive intellect reigned supreme to conspire with unbridled drives in an insane world of ruthless mutual manipulation for personal and political ends. The film characters with their clever lunatic smirks on their faces and the glint in their eyes showed the irretrievable loss of their humanity as they were compelled toward the ultimate goal of power, security, and pleasure—subject, of course, to the dictates of someone else's hidden power, security, and pleasure. The brutal murders, beatings, mutilations, mass rapes, and joyless orgies exhibited in that movie gave us a horrifying glimpse into the unavoidable mental states awaiting us a little further down the road.

Actually, that state has already arrived in sporadic form with the Bronx gangs, the bands of roving students attacking subway passengers in New York, and the "granny bashers" of London, girl bands who attack old people for robbery or fun.

What can account for our increasingly insane societal behavior? Why are people destroying each other—and caring so little that they are doing so?

In order for a thief to steal goods, the victim must not really exist as a person to him—only as an obstacle to the goods at hand, the only thing considered to have any validity at all. While the victim may find it a revealing and upsetting experience that "someone should do this to me," that someone should declare him personally invalid, he must remember that what prompted the thief to steal from him in the first place was a feeling of his *own* worthlessness. If the thief finds himself invalid and of no consequence in our world picture, he has nothing to lose except the pseudo-existence he believes he gains through illicit possessions.

It is our own intellectual world view's invalidation of man that has created social havoc. Muggers, robbers, killers, vandals, and rapists are not really interested in harming others; they are simply taking the invalidation of themselves and others to its final consequences. Intellect has no place for feelings, morals, and conscience; goods and their control, acquired in whatever "objective" way without emotional interference, are really what counts.

Rising criminality is only science made visible while feelings, concerns, and conscience are abolished as a valid human-social force. This is why the invalidation of man, while being declared "neutral"—which in human terms means amoral—is, in fact, the most immoral mental act in our mental history. Personal morality can find a true basis only in one's own sense of validity and value, and this is impossible in our totally intellectualized society.

If we are to curb crime and build a healthy, safe society, we must deview intellectual, depersonalized man. We must cease our delusional self-denial and accept and affirm our own being and that of others.

This new view incorporating the personal validity of man will lead to a genuine, mentally healthy atmosphere and, in turn, an open, trusting, mutually helpful society—the high mark of high culture.

The deep personal invalidation that has jeopardized the very principles of honesty, confidence, and love will progressively change into a more realistic recognition of people's unique value and being. As increasing numbers of people acquire a deeper sense of human value, the degree of temptation necessary to elicit dishonesty, distrust, or hate will rise. As the threshold rises, crime, suspicion, and social hostility that are now epidemic and still growing can be expected to subside. The basic mental cause—human invalidation—will have been eliminated.

Deviewing Intellectualized Man

Intellect continuously strives to make us a mere aspect of nature. Nature itself can afford to be amoral and nonhuman, for it has no purpose of its own. Nature simply perpetuates itself, with the *products* of nature constantly being destroyed by the *forces* of nature. But man is not only a product; by virtue of his mental faculties he is also a *force.* If man lives exclusively as a product of nature, as intellect would have him, he becomes a destructive element of nature.

Intellect professes to be objective, amoral, and neutral. But man himself cannot be any of these things and still be human. In addition, intellect's inability to deal with feelings and conscience allows unchecked drives to enter motives and purposes. Conscious amorality then turns into unconscious immorality. Human considerations, suffering, or life itself become *coincidental.* In purely intellectual thinking, human destruction would be removed from any moral judgment just as we do not judge one animal eating another in the world of nature. Intellect itself would express no judgment on Watergate, "mercy killing," or, for that matter, cannibalism, for man is really beside the point. But it would provide the know-how if for some external reason, in an emergency, for expediency, or plain efficiency, they were to be practiced. Intellect, then, is not only an incomplete way of looking at man; it is a dangerous one.

We must deview intellectualized man, realizing that intellectualism defines only part of man's existence. Intellect is a powerful mental tool, but as far as man goes it should always be mastered by our consciousness and not allowed to drift off unchecked into an inhuman, amoral world, taking passive man along with it.

If we deview intellectualized man and restore him to his full, human identity, we will avoid scientific "advances" and utopian schemes that attempt to advance man as a thing. No longer will we invent medical technology that simply prolongs external existence, creating vegetables of people whose illnesses have destroyed anything human left in them. Nor will we promulgate political and economic ideas whose primary concern is to have man become an efficient part of some larger system.

A new view of man would recognize the meaning and false lure of the many intellectual dreams (or nightmares) now come true and reject these, as well as those about to arrive on the scene. Even now, people proclaim "teaching machines are coming," or "psychotechnology is coming." Yet *must* they come, and if so, what is the *human* reason for them?

Brave New World is no further away than the completion of our intellectualized world picture. If we are to avoid Aldous Huxley's nightmare, we must reject the totally intellectual picture of things and put man back at the center of our world. Only then will we have a society that is truly a utopia, a society that is run on the basis of what is best for each full-blooded, individual human being.

Deviewing Intellectualized Thought, Feeling, and Will

The key to an intellectualized mind is *passivity.* Thinking, having come to mean little more than a mere reflection on "facts," loses its ability as an active, living mental force. Feeling becomes a mere response action. And as we limit ourselves to just responding, our own genuine emotional initiatives dry up, offering even less to respond to. This leads us into emotional starvation and subjects us to the far easier and almost "automatic" frustrated responses of *selfishness, hate, and fear.* And while unchecked drives run rampant, we have very little will left at all, our actions being nothing more than passive responses to intellect's conditioning.

This passivity of thought, feeling, and will is at the root of our mental health problems. We can no longer place faith in drugs that give us an illusion of mental health, or depend on the psychiatrists or friends of kindred heart who would listen to our problems to make us well again. We must learn first to reconstitute and then to strengthen our total selves on our own power. Only through the rebulding and mastering of all our mental abilities will we make ourselves whole and mentally healthy again.

1: The Management of Thinking Mobile, interpretive, creative universal thoughts require one's own initiative. The first goal in reconstituting our faculties must involve the reintroduction of our will into the sequence of our thoughts.

Intellect provided a sequence dictated passively by physical objects. It is one of the supreme delusions of science that these dictated sequences are "objectively" handled, when they are in reality subject to the unconsciously selective emotional choices of the scientist.

Brain science, for instance, moves mostly along paths of brain wave and metabolic research. That avenue is an emotional choice of scientists, because it conforms to their available instruments and gives them the greatest comfort in terms of method as well as "scientific" prestige.

We must make all thoughts our *own* thoughts—not those dictated by the inner laws of matter or our unconscious desires. *The conscious command over thought needs to be regained.*

Exercises in self-induced thinking can help us gain mastery over our thoughts. One such method is to take any object—a pencil, or a sheet of paper—and pursue a line of conscious thought about it: a description of the object, enumeration of its uses, the steps taken in its creation, and so on. Where one line of thought is exhausted, another one related to the same object should be chosen and pursued with equal concentration. Each thought needs to be pursued step by step to the end of its logical sequence. The essence of this exercise is the complete control of a continuing sequence of thought.

2: The Recovery of Feeling Mental reconstitution in the area of feeling involves *reintroduction of our will into our feelings, in order to lead us to improved mastery of our emotional life.*

What people believe to be spontaneous feelings are largely unfree, motivated unconsciously, or deceptive—and *negative.* They are no more spontaneous than the conditioning that usually created them. We must learn to gain control of our emotional life again, for to master feelings—and to create *positive* feelings—is the wellspring of mental health.

An exercise to help us do this is to find at least one attractive aspect in a person, thing, or event about which we feel negatively. This is no "moral" exercise, but an exercise of mental faculty. A simple resolution to become emotionally "objective" would be illusory, for that typical "objectivity" is nothing more than the prejudiced response founded by our intellect. To force ourselves to detect and appreciate a positive aspect that every being, object, or event may possess is to wrestle with our emotion to bring a new impersonal reality into our habitually subjective feelings.

The feelings that intellect ridicules most contemptuously turn out to be the feelings usually elicited in these exercises. They are the most valuable and difficult of all: love, devotion, and trust. Here mental laws are truly at variance with physical laws. Here a true intellectual would cringe, for he could not grasp the law by which love fills the pouring cup and hate empties the receiving one. He could never understand how love in warming us needs no reason at all. Nor could he ever consider that devotion or dedication leads us to know more about the subject of our devotion than all the intellect in the world. Intellect could not follow us into the complete identification with the subject of our dedication by embracing its inner qualities, but stands back to measure the outer qualities alone.

This generation of positive feelings will help us countermand the automatic negative responses of selfishness, hate, and fear, which are the main forces of our mental disruption. Once we have done this, we are on our way back to mental health.

3: The Rebuilding of Will Strengthening will is a matter of *making decisions and carrying them out to the hilt, repetitively and regularly.*

These may be simple actions. One may decide to turn one's ring around at noon, or look at the sky to observe the clouds at 3 P.M. daily, or walk around a chair at 9 P.M. or set aside a daily time for a five-minute meditation, or tear a page out of a daily calendar before going to bed. What counts is a decision that results in completed action.

Difficulties in continuing the practice will test our ability to will. But after a time of consistent practice, perhaps several weeks, one will find that at the right time one no longer forgets even while in the middle of another quite absorbing task. The beginning of a new will that comes to life in our decisions now exhorts us to "*do* our thing."

Being decisions of our own, they have nothing to do with neurotic self-estranged compulsions that overwhelm what is left of our healthy will under pathological circumstances.

The making of decisions and their continuing enactment—regardless of purpose—strengthen our willpower just as continuing physical exercise—regardless of purpose—strengthens our musclepower. Through repetition, willpower, much like musclepower, can take on ever greater challenges to carry through initiatives. If life and mind live *in* action willpower *is* the power within the action. It is the strengthening of one's own will that will make the action our own.

Proof that decisions and their repetitive enactment strengthen will is that they alleviate depression—the paralysis of will marked by withdrawal, lack of initiative, and low spirits, in deadlocked anger-fear situations. They do so because a new mastery appeases our fears and a new confidence soothes our anger.

A nationwide epidemic of mental disorder has been brought about by an intellect-drenched world view that blunts our thinking, controls our feelings, and paralyzes our will. When we once again have control of these precious mental abilities, we will have a truly modern mentally healthy culture. Our mental health will no longer depend on the humanly empty promises of the physical sciences, or on technology that is itself a creation of the self-estranged shadows of "technological man." It will depend upon *whole man,* who will use the mental faculties he has regained to gain mastery once again over his world.

The Value of Consciousness as the Basis for Mental Health

Intellect, science, and technology have grown destructive to our mental health not on their own account, but by default because our consciousness failed to gain an overview and use them as helpers in human development. It is therefore obvious that consciousness will be increasingly essential for our mental health in the future.

We must once again become conscious of some basic mental health principles. Certain principles of mental health have always been applied unconsciously, but they have gradually faded under the onslaught of intellect. Mental health principles are simply truths that our mind takes for granted, as if inherent in its very nature. Conscious or unconscious, the mind lives by them, and they form the basis for our mental health. They are typically "unthinkable," denied, or ignored by intellect, as they are entirely incongruent with our world picture. These principles, so crucial to our mental health, are the following: *permanence, inner freedom, activity, growth, essentiality, hierarchy of being, and the feeling of belonging on one's terms.*

Permanence is the feeling that no matter what else in life appears elusive or empty, the human mind—the very essence of self—is a permanent reality. The deeper entrenched we are intellectually, the more repressed this principle becomes—the more life appears empty, and the more we search for substitute meanings. Regardless of what intellect may declare, the mind has made up its mind about its own permanence, and it demonstrates this in all its actions throughout life.

Inner freedom is an ability to do things out of our very own being, and not as induced by self-estranged forces within us. This is a key principle of mental health.

Mental activity and mental growth are the very life of the mind. Also, we must feel that we have mastery over the mind, that we ourselves are what is giving it direction, and that it is always advancing. If we are not masters of our own minds, the mind will not be our reality—it will only be busy, slipping from our command to serve other real or illusory determinants. When this happens, carried to its extreme it means *insanity.* Growth is important, too, for standstill to the mind means anguish, regression, and existential loss, inasmuch as it is an intrinsic need of the mind to have a definite sense of growth into a more meaningful future.

Essentiality is the ability to see the permanent "self" in all human beings. Thoughts, feelings, and impulses are constantly changing, disappearing, and reappearing in new forms, yet each person maintains a continuous, essential quality that is derived from the self. To the extent that it is healthy, the mind will instinctively remain attuned to the "permanent" essentiality of people that emanates from their self.

Awareness of the hierarchy of being allows us to see the relative importance of things. Intellect has us dealing with all truths on one level, ignoring the comprehensive laws of hierarchal truth. It thinks nothing of observing a specimen of some human organ on a microscopic slide and then making pronouncements about the whole nature of man or the destiny of a culture. If we restore the mental health principle of hierarchically interrelating meanings, we will really restore mental health, for mental health means an *accurate, authentic relationship to meanings.*

The last mental health principle, that of "belonging," concerns the absolute requirement of a healthy mind to interrelate and to belong—and the equally urgent requirement of the modern mind to do so as a unique, self-determining entity. Here individualism creates elbow room to test man's ability to be free, independent, and spontaneous in his relationships, which is to say *conscious* in his relationships. Belonging with people is an obvious mental necessity; to belong and to live on one's terms is a mental health principle required in our time.

To be conscious of these mental health principles and to apply them will have a mentally invigorating effect on each one of us. To know through consciousness is indeed the supreme mental health principle.

Consciousness lives in relationships, relationships of concepts, ideas, events, and people. Intellect is the obsession with difference exclusive of relationship and meaning.

For the purpose of restoring our mental health, much would be gained if a degree of consciousness of self, self-consciousness, a consciousness as whole human beings within a universe of multilevel realities, could become an individual and cultural characteristic of ours. And even more—infinitely more—in terms of mental health and human development could be secured if we would move on from our spuriously "objective" intellectualizations to *objective consciousness,* a supreme mental-spiritual goal where the comprehensive realities our consciousness gathers could be grasped as objective truth. It is in such ways, and in such ways only, that we will restore our mental health and build a freer, happier, healthier society.

The Value of Consciousness as a Method cf Knowledge

We believe we have a method to understand matter, but we have no method to understand life itself, and while intellect alone may be able to explain how a machine runs, it has consistently failed to explain matters of life, mind, and spirit. Only a new method that reaches far beyond the limited scientific view can explain these things.

Several have tried. Johann Wolfgang von Goethe endeavored to find a method to understand life where it is found in its purest, simplest form—in plants. Believing that the laboratory procedure of analysing life's dead products was not adequate, Goethe instead worked by means of thought as orderly, living, and real as the plants he tried to fathom. He came to recognize an archetype, a living force-entity that was present in all plants. The principles of metamorphosis, of contraction and expansion, and of rhythm in time and space that *are nature to any plant* were the visible expressions of this living entity. Goethe actually viewed his archetype as a living reality and the idea of it as a living idea that could grasp the living plant.

Goethe made the first serious attempt in history to create a methodology of consciousness, a valid means of universal thought that required unaccustomed mental effort far beyond intellect's passive observation and measurement. Naturally, then, it was totally ignored.

Current opinion also denies that there could be any method to understand life itself, much less mind or spirit. Behaviorism, for instance, has solved the problem by denying their existence, and in all other walks of life spiritual matters are as a matter of course relegated to the domain of mere belief.

The most stringent and reliable methods today that attempt to penetrate these vast uncharted areas of life, mind, and spirit are those given us by Rudolf Steiner, the founder of a worldwide system of child and adult education in the first quarter of this century. Steiner built a methodology that explored man himself through new mental abilities developed in full consciousness and in a systematic manner. Progressing from fully controlled thinking to self-generated living thinking, to "imaginative cognition," to "inspiration," and "intuition"—all well-defined levels of advancing cognition—the difficulty and validity of these methods far exceed those used in today's science.

Steiner's method of consciousness is relatively unknown, not because it lacks scientific rigor but because it does not conform to the attitudes upheld by our present world view. His method when applied offers truly human solutions in such fields as science, education, medicine, and the arts, but they, too, have been largely ignored on the authority of conditioned preferences parading as science in our time.

The greatest opportunity to explore our world and solve its problems can only come through the development of that consciousness which has lain dormant for so long. Until we do this, the rusty gates of intellect will continue to hold us prisoners, removed not only from the luminous reality our thoughts could have, but also from the vast universe of the spiritual realities that could be encompassed with our rational mind.

Where from Here?

Time is running out. A four-hundred-year-old world conception has reduced man to purely physical properties. It has gradually become a science and is now a way of life that destroys him. We can no longer subsist on binges of nostalgia and self-reassuring pretenses, for man is now in the process of losing his will to be human.

Something must be done—and soon. But preaching, writing theses, and announcing statistical, computerized research findings are not going to bring about any real changes in human affairs. They cannot, for they themselves are a creation of the sick mentality that got us into this unhealthy personal and societal state in the first place. That sick mentality is intellect, and any intellectual suggestions for change will only be anachronistic, mind-disabling, manipulative, or coercive.

Mental recovery today must literally be built on the creation of *new* mental foundations—the validity of the individual, his creation of himself as a living reality, and the perception of everyone else on earth as equally valid and real. It depends on seeing the world this way in ever smaller daily details.

It is this change of view, based on new insights, that

alone can bring a change in ourselves: in how we see ourselves, how we see others, what we consider to be our life's purposes, and what we tolerate or do not tolerate of others in these new contexts.

It will be a mental change that raises us to a level of experience of our being that has been virtually lost along with our mental stability. That will be the change *within.* If it occurs in sufficient numbers of people, it must inevitably lead to crucial social changes. The mental self-assurance derived from this self-affirmation will see improving mental health, a new morality based on mental principles acknowledged in liberty, and new spontaneous man-concerned attitudes that will make for social peace and progress. It will mean a new *human*-oriented world, the *only* kind of world that is truly able to sustain human beings in their full human potential. Time is indeed running out, and if we are to save ourselves from a depersonalized mechanistic oblivion, we must again grasp what is real inside us. We must once again remind ourselves that *we are human*—and *that is everything.*

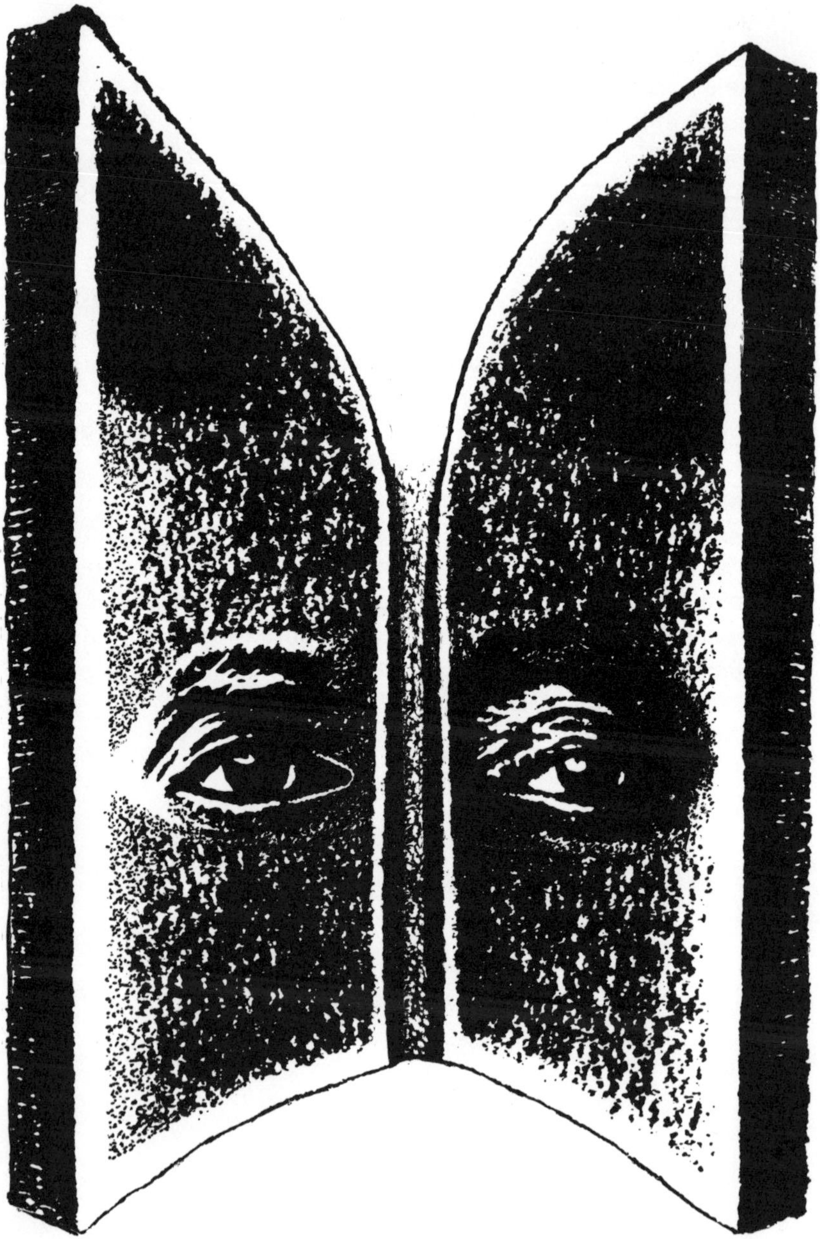

NOTES

Introduction

[1] Based on latest data obtained from the National Institute of Mental Health Biometry Department, September, 1972. These figures are to be considered estimates owing to the number of undiagnosed, inaccessible, or borderline cases.

[2] Ibid.

[3] Group for the Advancement of Psychiatry, *Basic Considerations in Mental Retardation: A Preliminary Report* (December, 1959), p. 8.

[4] *Alcohol and Health,* First Special Report to Congress from the Secretary of Health, Education and Welfare (HSM 72–9099), 1971, p. vi.

[5] Based on latest data obtained from the NIMH Biometry Department, September, 1972.

[6] HEW Report on National Health of 1962, released 1972; Leo Schrole, Thomas S. Langner, Stanley T. Michael, Marvin K. Opler, Thomas A. Rennie, *Mental Health in the Metropolis, the Midtown Manhattan Study* (New York: McGraw Hill, 1962), p. 138.

[7] In 1969, a Manhattan study rated 88 percent of children as having some type of mental disturbance. Of these 42 percent showed mild disturbance, 34 percent moderate, 11 percent marked, and 1 percent severe impairment (Thomas S. Langner, et al., "Economic and Ethnic Differences in Psychiatric Impairment in a Random Sample of Urban Children," *American Journal of Orthopsychiatry,* Vol. 39, 1969). In studies of suburbia, children did not fare any better. In Westchester, N.Y., for instance, professional intervention was thought to be required for 55 to 60 percent of children. Generally a vast majority of children from all economic and sociocultural backgrounds—our next generation—"appeared to be anxious, confused, had low self-esteem, poor motivation, problems of impulse control, and pervasive feelings of discontent." (Olga R. Lurie, *The Emotional Health of Children in the Family Setting,* published by the Mental Health Association of Westchester County, July 1, 1970.)

I. The Man-made Century

[1] Telegram addressed to the Commissioner of the New York City Department of Mental Health and Mental Retardation Services, May 16, 1972, signed by the Coordinating Committee of Employee Organizations.

[2] Rand Corporation study requested for the New York City Department of Mental Health and Mental Retardation Services, 1970.

[3] Information obtained in 1972 from the New York City deputy medical examiner.

[4] William Nebel, as cited by Alvin Toffler in *Future Shock* (New York: Random House, 1970), p. 77.

[5] Joint Commission on Mental Health of Children, Inc., *Digest of Crisis in Child Mental Health: Challenge for the 1970's* (Washington, D.C.: Joint Commission on Mental Health of Children, Inc., 1969), p. 6.

[6] Ibid., p. 28.

[7] Based on interviews with patients.

[8] Based on interviews with patients.

[9] Based on interviews with patients.

[10] Malachi Martin, "The Scientist as Shaman," *Harper's Magazine* (March, 1972), p. 59.

II. The School: An Education in Insanity

[1] Based on interview with a student.

[2] Daniel Hauben, "Diary," in Ronald Gross and Paul Osterman, eds., *High School* (New York: Simon & Schuster, 1971), p. 92.

[3] Based on interviews with students.

[4] Montgomery County Student Alliance, "Wanted: A Humane Education," in Gross and Osterman, *High School,* p. 108.

[5] Daniel Hauben, in Gross and Osterman, *High School,* p. 107.

[6] Ibid., p. 87.

[7] "Grades, Bah Humbug!!" by *The Open Door* (a student newspaper), Milwaukee, Wis., in Gross and Osterman, *High School*, p. 156.

[8] Based on interview with a student.

[9] Elizabeth M. Eddy, "Discipline Classes in Urban School," *Walk the White Line, a Profile of Urban Education* (New York: Anchor Books, 1967).

[10] Based on interview with a student.

[11] Based on interviews with students.

[12] William C. Morse, "The Mental Hygiene Viewpoint on School Discipline," in Harvey F. Clarizio, ed., *Mental Health and the Educative Process* (New York: Rand McNally & Co., 1969).

[13] Kathryn J. Noyes and Gordon L. McAndrew, "Is This What Schools Are For?" *Saturday Review* (December 21, 1968).

[14] Charles E. Silberman, *Crisis in the Classroom* (New York: Random House, 1970), p. 182.

[15] Patricia Minuchin, Barbara Biber, Edna Shapiro, and Herbert Zimiles, *The Psychological Impact of School Experience* (New York: Basic Books, Inc., 1969), p. 408.

[16] Lawrence Stolurow, as cited by Silberman, *Crisis in the Classroom*, p. 195.

[17] Anthony G. Oettinger, as cited by Silberman, *Crisis in the Classroom*, p. 192.

[18] Robert Glaser, discussion of Oettinger and Mark's "Educational Technology: New Myths and Old Realities," in *Harvard Educational Review*, vol. 38, no. 4 (Fall 1968), as cited by Silberman, *Crisis in the Classroom*, pp. 197–198.

[19] Patrick Suppes, "The Use of Computers in Education," *Scientific American* (September, 1966).

[20] Robert Glaser, as cited by Silberman, *Crisis in the Classroom*, p. 200.

III. Technology: Destructive Intellect Unleashed

[1] Roger Starr, as cited by Glenn Collins in "Notes on a Revolutionary Dinosaur," *The New York Times Magazine* (August 6, 1972), p. 31.

[2] Richard G. Stein, as cited by Glenn Collins, "Notes on a Revolutionary Dinosaur," p. 24.

[3] Jacques Ellul, *The Technological Society* (New York: Alfred A. Knopf, Inc., 1964), p. 421.

[4] Ibid., p. 334.

[5] Ibid., p. 139.

[6] James McKeen Cattell, as cited by Loren Baritz in "The Servants of Power," in Jack D. Douglas, ed., *Freedom and Tyranny: Social Problems in a Technological Society* (New York: Alfred A. Knopf, Inc., 1970), p. 197.

[7] Facts and quotes in this paragraph as cited by Loren Baritz, "Servants of Power," pp. 208–209.

[8] R. L. Tobin, "This Program May Be Harmful to Your Child," *Saturday Review* (October 9, 1971).

[9] Ibid.

[10] "T.V. Violence: 'Appalling,' " *U.S. News & World Report* (October 6, 1969).

[11] T. Berry Brazelton, as cited in "T.V.: A Wasteland for Tots," *Christian Century* (April 26, 1972).

[12] Gerald Looney, as cited in "T.V.: A Wasteland for Tots."

IV. Man's Changing View of Himself: How Man's Humanity Was Lost

[1] Galileo Galilei, as cited by Lewis Mumford, *The Myth of the Machine, The Pentagon of Power* (New York: Harcourt Brace Jovanovich, Inc. 1970), p. 61.

[2] Ibid., p. 79.

V. Modern Psychology and the Loss of Reality

[1] John B. Watson, *Behaviorism* (New York: W. W. Norton & Co., 1930), p. 3.

[2] Ibid., p. 6.

[3] B. F. Skinner, *Beyond Freedom and Dignity* (New York: Alfred A. Knopf, 1971), pp. 125, 200–201.

[4] C. G. Jung, *Psychological Types,* translated by H. G. Barnes (New York: Harcourt, Brace, 1923).